Ethel Chehter
Alexandre Barbosa

AIDS and Pancreas in the HAART Era: A Cross Sectional Study

AF138626

Ethel Chehter
Alexandre Barbosa

AIDS and Pancreas in the HAART Era:
A Cross Sectional Study

LAP LAMBERT Academic Publishing

Impressum / Imprint

Bibliografische Information der Deutschen Nationalbibliothek: Die Deutsche Nationalbibliothek verzeichnet diese Publikation in der Deutschen Nationalbibliografie; detaillierte bibliografische Daten sind im Internet über http://dnb.d-nb.de abrufbar.
Alle in diesem Buch genannten Marken und Produktnamen unterliegen warenzeichen-, marken- oder patentrechtlichem Schutz bzw. sind Warenzeichen oder eingetragene Warenzeichen der jeweiligen Inhaber. Die Wiedergabe von Marken, Produktnamen, Gebrauchsnamen, Handelsnamen, Warenbezeichnungen u.s.w. in diesem Werk berechtigt auch ohne besondere Kennzeichnung nicht zu der Annahme, dass solche Namen im Sinne der Warenzeichen- und Markenschutzgesetzgebung als frei zu betrachten wären und daher von jedermann benutzt werden dürften.

Bibliographic information published by the Deutsche Nationalbibliothek: The Deutsche Nationalbibliothek lists this publication in the Deutsche Nationalbibliografie; detailed bibliographic data are available in the Internet at http://dnb.d-nb.de.
Any brand names and product names mentioned in this book are subject to trademark, brand or patent protection and are trademarks or registered trademarks of their respective holders. The use of brand names, product names, common names, trade names, product descriptions etc. even without a particular marking in this works is in no way to be construed to mean that such names may be regarded as unrestricted in respect of trademark and brand protection legislation and could thus be used by anyone.

Coverbild / Cover image: www.ingimage.com

Verlag / Publisher:
LAP LAMBERT Academic Publishing
ist ein Imprint der / is a trademark of
OmniScriptum GmbH & Co. KG
Heinrich-Böcking-Str. 6-8, 66121 Saarbrücken, Deutschland / Germany
Email: info@lap-publishing.com

Herstellung: siehe letzte Seite /
Printed at: see last page
ISBN: 978-3-659-61382-1

Copyright © 2014 OmniScriptum GmbH & Co. KG
Alle Rechte vorbehalten. / All rights reserved. Saarbrücken 2014

Alexandre Gutierre Barbosa

Ethel Zimberg Chehter

AIDS and Pancreas in the HAART Era: A Cross Sectional Study.

2012

Dedication

People with HIV who believe in scientific research in order to alleviate the symptoms of the disease and strengthen the hope of healing.

Acknowledgments

Firstly to God, for giving me the privilege of doing this work.

To my parents, for always being present in every step of my life, providing security, protection, dialogue, affection and love.

To my sister, who has always believed in me, in all times.

To my advisor Dr. Ethel Zimberg Chehter, MD, PhD, AGAF, who I very much admire, for her dedication and professionalism in carrying out this work. An example to be followed.

To Dr. Ana Maria Mader, MD, PhD, for her dedication and professionalism in microscopic slides analysis. It has been an honor to have you on the team.

To Dr. Sonia Malheiros Lopes Sanioto, PhD, for the supporting my persistence in science and for believing in my professional capacity. Thank you for being my guide in the course of Physiology, in Faculdade de Medicina do ABC (FMABC).

To Juan, laboratory technician of the Pathology Department of FMABC, for his talent in the preparations of the microscopic slides, his dedication, carefulness and esteem.

Table of Contents

1. INTRODUCTION

1.1 OVERVIEW

AIDS is a pandemic disease that affects over 34 million people worldwide [1]. In Brazil there are around 590,000 infected individuals, with a higher concentration of cases in the state of São Paulo - 344,150 - followed by the southern region of the country, with a total of 115,598 cases [2].

According to the literature, until the year 2000 pancreatic involvement in HIV patients varied from 11 to 65%. However, the majority of studies are retrospective with histological data rarely reported [3,4,5,6]. We found no systematic prospective study of pancreatic disease in AIDS reported in the literature.

The pancreatic changes in patients infected with HIV may be due to causes unrelated to AIDS, such as alcoholism, diabetes, cholelithiasis, adenocarcinoma, acute pancreatitis, chronic pancreatitis and medications [5,6,7,8,9]. On the other hand, causes related to AIDS include opportunistic infections and drugs used in its treatment, such as asparaginase and azathioprine among others [5-9].

A study conducted by Chehter [5] in 2000 found pancreatic abnormalities in patients who had died of AIDS without antiretroviral treatment due to protein-caloric malnutrition. The possible causes for these alterations were: malnutrition, weight loss and wasting syndrome. The wasting syndrome associated factors found in this study were: anorexia, dysphagia, odynophagia, medications, neurological factors, diarrhea, pancreatic enzyme deficiency, increased muscle protein, hyper metabolism and increase of cytokines. The microscopic histological aspects revealed decrease in the zymogen granules in the pancreatic acinar cells, parenchymal atrophy, steatosis and nuclear alterations represented by pyknosis, double layered, irregularly shaped at times, namely "dysplasia-like" [5, 6]. These findings may suggest that a pancreas with such characteristics could generate clinical-laboratorial alterations, indicating exocrine pancreatic insufficiency. These facts could only be better understood with the knowledge of antiviral effects.

The current study establishes a comparative analysis of the pancreatic histology in patients who in 1995 died of AIDS without HAART (High Active Antiretroviral Therapy) and in those who in 2010 died of the same cause under the use of this therapy.

1.2 HISTORY

The first reported cases on AIDS date from 1981 among young homosexuals in the United States. Today, however, the idea that disease cases had occurred four years before it was firstly identified is widely accepted [10].

Back then it was described as a syndrome characterized by a deep immune suppression with many clinical aspects which included opportunistic infections, malignant diseases and the central nervous system degeneration [10,11].

In 1984 American and French researchers simultaneously identified the retrovirus HIV in cells of patients with AIDS, and from that moment on it has been considered the etiologic agent of the disease [10].

After a long feud, the primacy of the French scientists from the Pasteur Institute over the American researchers regarding the identification of the HIV virus was acknowledged [10].

Despite the fact the virus's origin is still unknown, one of the hypotheses is that it arose in Central Africa as an indirect mutant form of a non-pathogenic virus found in the monkey *Cercopithecus aethiops* [10].

There are two genetically different but related forms of HIV isolated in patients with AIDS: HIV-1 and HIV-2. The former is the most common type associated with AIDS in the United States, Europe and Central Africa whereas the latter causes a similar disease, especially in Western Africa. In 1986 HIV-2 was detected in Lisbon in individuals who came from Guinea-Bissau and Cape Verde, Portuguese islands located off the coast of Western Africa [10,11,12]. Later on, the virus was found in six European countries. It is extremely rare in the United States [13].

HIV-1 and HIV-2 are similarly transmitted; however, HIV-2 high-risk groups are individuals who work as sex professionals and those with other sexually transmitted diseases [10,11,14].

1.3 EPIDEMIOLOGY

Since the infection by the HIV was established in humans, its proliferation has been boosted by multiple factors. The advent of quick air travel in the 20th century provided a means of the virus spread [14].

Urbanization led to an increase in number of infected people owing to their promiscuous sexual behaviors with partners from all over the world. Moreover, the introduction and distribution of new I.V. drugs were made easier [1,15].

The AIDS pandemic has evolved over time. Four main stages of evolution can be identified [14]: in the beginning the virus broke out from endemic species in rural areas and spread among urban populations; in the second stage propagation occurred due to risk behaviors, including sexual promiscuity and the use of I.V. drugs, which led to the third stage throughout the 1980s when the infection rate quickly increased in the United States; the fourth stage occurred in some regions like Western Europe, North America and Australia where control measures were taken with positive effects. Nevertheless, in some areas like Central Africa and Asia the epidemic rates kept rising throughout the 1990s and the 21st century [1,14,15].

By the end of the 20th century, over 21 million people worldwide had died of AIDS; over 34 million people were infected with the HIV virus, and among this total, 95% of the individuals had been living in developing countries. In the antiretroviral therapy era in the United States, the median life expectancy of people who were infected with the virus increased from 10.5 years in 1996 to 22.5 years in 2005 [1,15].

The most affected age group is youngsters aged between 15 - 24 years, representing 40% of new infection cases. All over the world, more than 50% of the infected patients are women, and one of the consequences is the perinatal infection resulting in a significant number of children born infected with HIV [11,14].

1.4 CURRENT STATE OF THE HIV EPIDEMICS

According to UNAIDS, the Joint United Nations Programme on HIV/AIDS, there are around 33.4 million people infected by the HIV virus in the world. Among this total, around 5.7 million individuals live in South Africa, which makes it the leading country in number of cases of HIV carriers [1].

In the United States, there are around 1.1 million infected individuals according to the Centers for Disease Control and Prevention (CDC). About 20% of homo- or bisexual men who live in big cities are HIV carriers. After conducting a survey in 21 major cities in the USA in the year 2010, the CDC revealed that this rate rises to 28% among black men, a much greater number of cases when compared with white (16%) or Asian (8%) men. Among the cities the survey encompassed, Baltimore had the highest rate of HIV prevalence (38%), followed by New York (29%), Dallas and Houston (26%) and Miami (25%) [13].

The latest MOH Epidemiological News Bulletin from 2010 reports that Latin America registers 1.4 million infected individuals, and that 0.5% of the total Brazilian population is an HIV carrier. Since the beginning of the epidemics 20 years ago, 590 thousand Brazilians have been infected, and within this amount 150 thousand have died [15].

The number of AIDS cases in Brazil is higher among males. From 1980 to June 2010 a total of 385,815 infection cases in males and 207,080 cases in females were registered (65.1% vs. 34.9%) according to the same bulletin mentioned above. It also states an increase of the disease among women, especially homemakers, in the last months of 2010. As a result, the Ministry of Health has been mentioning the feminization of the disease since the difference in number of cases between males and females is getting smaller and smaller. The number of cases among youngsters aged between 13 and 19 years increased, and only in this age group is the number of female AIDS cases higher [15].

According to the Brazilian MOH bulletin on AIDS and Sexually Transmitted Diseases, the highest concentration of infected individuals is in the Southeast, with 344,150 cases (58%), followed by the South, with 115,598 cases (19.5%), the Northeast, with 74,364 cases (12.5%), the Center-West, with 34,057 cases (5.7%) and the North, with 24,745 cases (4.2%) [15].

It is in the South, however, where the highest incidence rate is reported, with a total of 32.4 cases for every 100 thousand inhabitants, followed by the Southeast (20.4), the North (20.1), the Center-West (18) and the Northeast (13.9). The data show that most HIV carriers in Brazil in the year 2010 were white (47.7%), followed by black individuals (46.8%), yellow individuals (0.5%) and native Brazilians (0.3%). A total of 4.7% individuals did not define their race or color [15].

The bulletin also reveals that the antiretroviral therapy increased life expectancy in HIV-positive patients from 7% in 2003 to 42% in 2008. Despite the fact the rapid expansion of access to the therapy has been decreasing mortality rates related to AIDS since 2010, the high cost of the treatment is still a major hindrance. Pharmaceutical multinationals still sell medications to governments at sky-high prices [15].

2. HIV

HIV virion has a diameter of around 120 nm, and the electron microscopic images show a dense cylindrical core surrounded by a lipid layer with two glycoproteins, **gp120** and **gp41**, forming **gp160** complexes; right below it there is a layer, the virus matrix **p17** protein, which encloses the capsid to maintain the integrity of the viral particle [5,10,11,12,14,17].

The capsid is composed of approximately 2,000 copies of the viral protein **p24**, and the genetic material is made of two molecules of RNA, reverse transcriptase **p66** and **p51** and proteins **p9** and **p6** [5,10,11,12,14].

The HIV genome (RNA) is tightly bound to the nucleocapsid proteins **p7**, **p55**, **p40** and **p24**.

The HIV genome contains three major genes: **Gag (polyprotein processed by viral protease)**, **Pol (Polymerase)** and **Env (gp160 protein of the virus capsule)**. They contain the necessary information to make new viral particles from the structural and functional proteins of the HIV virus [5,10,11,12,14,17].

The HIV core structure can be seen in cross section in **Figure 1** where the capsid structural protein and the bilipid layer with many associated glycoproteins are represented.

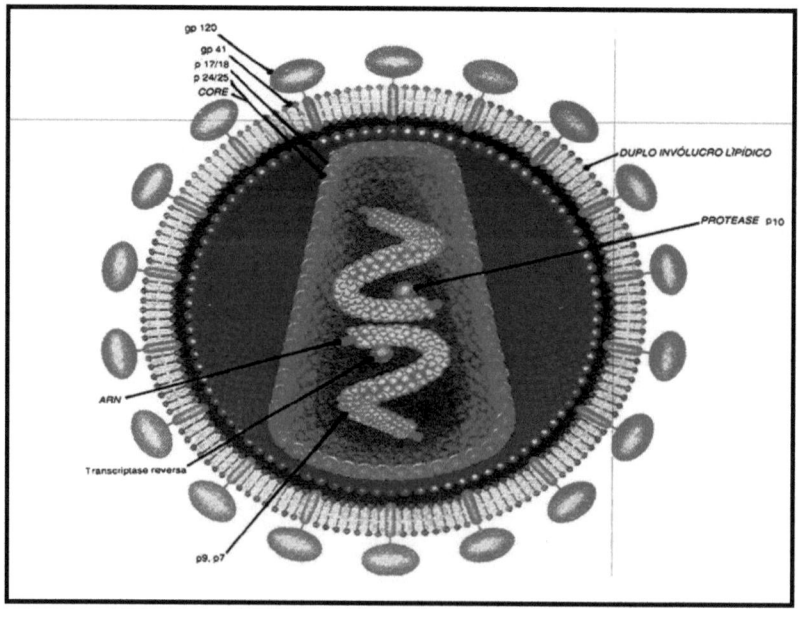

Figure 1 Scheme of HIV structure. Cross section showing the virus core with two strands of RNA and the enzyme reverse transcriptase, protease p10 and proteins p9 and p7 linked to them. The core envelope contains proteins p24, p25, p17 and p18. The virus is surrounded by a lipid bilayer originated from the host cell, binding the gp120 glycoprotein which, in turn, is anchored to the gp41. Other glycoproteins (gp110 and gp140) are found inside the buttons of the gp120 which form lipid bilayer. **Source**: [17].

2.1 VIROLOGY

CD4 molecule is the main receptor for the HIV virus on the cell surface along with the co-receptors **CCR5** and **CXCR4** [5,10,11,12,14]. It is expressed on the surface of T helper lymphocytes (**T-tropic**), macrophages (**M-tropic**), monocytes, follicular dendritic cells of lymph nodes and of the microglia, skin Langerhans cells, intestinal epithelial cells, uterine cervical cells (with little known clinical significance), natural killer (NK) cells, hematological precursors, vascular smooth muscle and fibroblasts can be infected by the HIV virus [5,10,11,12,14].

The HIV virus that only uses the **CCR5** co-receptor is called **R5**; the virus that only uses the **CXCR4** co-receptor is called **X4**; the virus that uses both co-receptors is called **X4R5** [5,10,11,12,14].

The chemokines (**CCR5** and **CXCR4** co-receptors) are powerful mediators or inflammatory regulators given their ability to recruit and activate specific leukocyte subpopulations. They are a big family of cytokines, structurally similar, that stimulate and regulate the migration of leukocytes from the blood to the tissues.

The M-tropic HIV strains interact with the **CCR5 (R5)** chemokine co-receptors to infect macrophages and dendritic cells. **CCR8** was identified as a co-receptor that allows the infection of not only T cells (lymphocytes), but also of M cells (macrophages). Throughout time, HIV mutations may increase the virus's capacity to infect cells via such pathways, starting with the predominance of **CCR5**-tropic virus strains. The T-tropic HIV strains interact with the **CXCR4 (X4)** co-receptors to infect lymphocytes. The alpha-chemokine **SDF1**, a ligand for **CXCR4** co-receptors, suppresses the replication of T-tropic viruses in order to regulate the **CXCR4** expression on the surface of these cells [5,10,11,12,14].

➢ The stages of HIV cell cycle can be described as follows:

• HIV viral entry into the host cell starts with the interaction of glycoproteins **gp120** and **gp41,** which form the glycoprotein **gp160.** It, in turn, binds to the specific cell surface receptor **CD4** with the help of the chemokine   co-receptors **CCR5** or **CXCR4**, allowing the N-terminal fusion peptide of gp41 to penetrate the cell membrane and releasing the virus core into the cytoplasm of the host cell [5,10,11,12,14]. **(Figure 2)**

Figure 2: The molecular basis of HIV entry into the cell. **Source** [16]

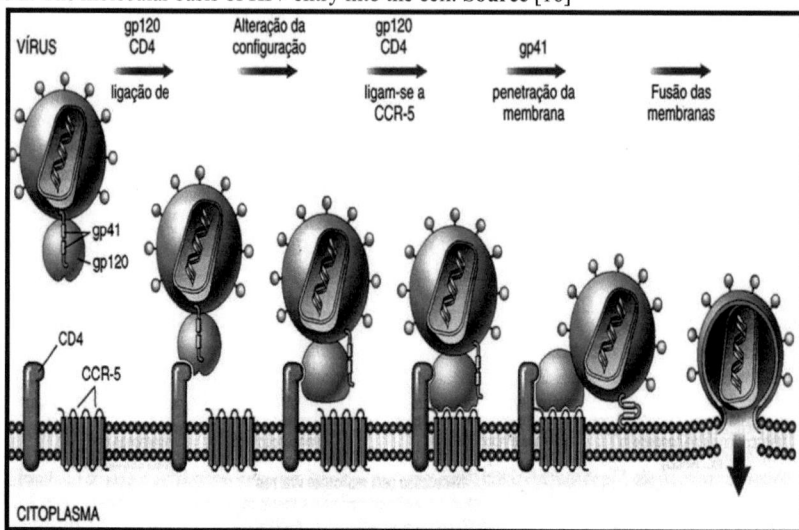

Figure 2: VIRUS - gp120/CD4 binding - Alteration in Configuration - gp120/CD4/bind to CCR5 - gp41/membrane penetration - Fusion of Membranes – Cytoplasm

The viral RNA is transcribed into complementary DNA through the enzyme reverse transcriptase. Next, the complementary DNA is transported to the cell nucleus through the enzyme integrase, favoring viral integration in the host cell genome and originating the provirus [5,10,11,12,14]. **(Figure 3)**

During the virus replication, the DNA (provirus) is transcribed into viral messenger RNA and moves to the cell cytoplasm, where viral proteins will be produced and broken down into subunits by the enzyme protease. Viral proteins will regulate the synthesis of new viral genomes and form the outer structure of other viruses that will be released by the host cell to the surrounding medium. They may either remain in the extracellular fluid or infect new cells [5,10,11,12,14] (Figure 3).

Figure 3 HIV life cycle. Illustration of the stages, from the entry of the virus into the host cell to the production of infectious virions. **Source** [16]

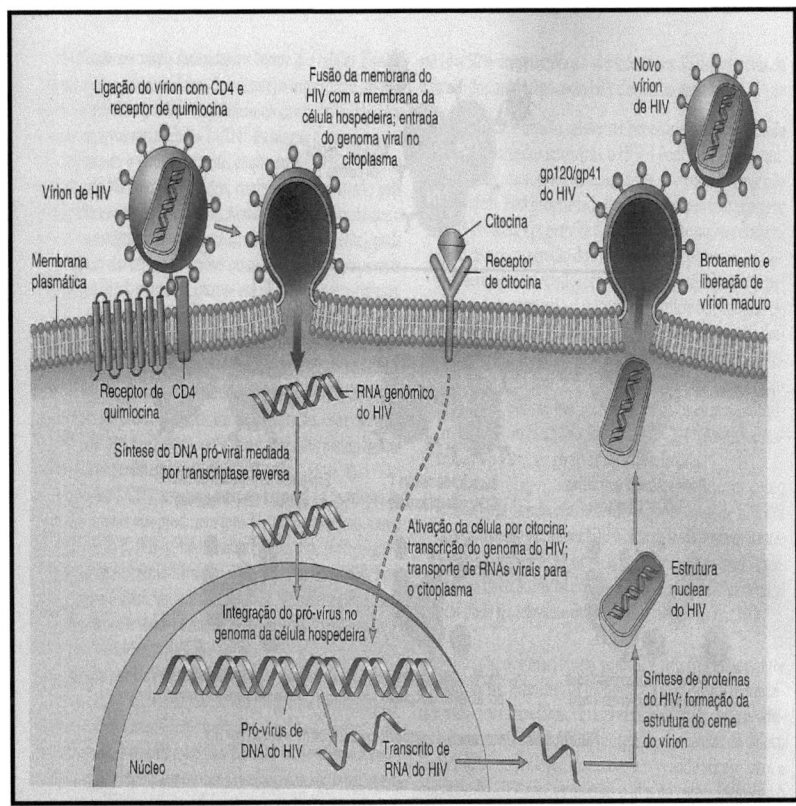

Figure 3 Plasmatic membrane - HIV virion - Virion binding to CD4 and chemokine receptor - Fusion of the host cell and the viral membranes; viral genome entry into cytoplasm - Cytokine and cytokine receptor - New HIV virion - HIV gp120/gp41- Budding and release of mature virion.

Chemokine receptor - CD4 - HIV genomic RNA - Proviral DNA synthesis mediated by reverse transcriptase - Cell activation by cytokine; HIV genome transcription; viral RNA transport to cytoplasm - Nuclear structure of HIV - Provirus integration into genome of host cell.

Nucleus - HIV proviral DNA - HIV RNA transcript - HIV protein synthesis, formation of the virion core structure.

3.   THE NATURAL HISTORY OF AIDS

The natural history of HIV infection may be divided into:

➢   Viral transmission;
➢   acute retroviral syndrome;
➢   seroconversion;
➢   clinical latency stage with or without persistent lymphadenopathy;
➢   early symptomatic HIV infection;
➢   AIDS.

The total sequence of events in an ordinary patient, in the absence of HIV treatment, takes around 10 years from seroconversion to death. Nearly 54% of the patients evolve to AIDS in 11 years. A summary of 20 reports revealed that the median time from seroconversion to AIDS is of 7 years in transfused patients, 10 years in hemophilic patients, 10 years in I.V. drug users and 8-12 years in male homosexuals. However, in a study conducted with patients who underwent medical treatment in an urban center, there was no difference in the disease progression or life expectancy that could be associated with sex, race, use of I.V. drugs or socioeconomic status. The age factor is related to an increased mortality rate. Patients over 35 years of age present median progression time to AIDS of 6 years whereas this median increases to 15 years in patients between 16 and 24 years of age. The median life expectancy after a CD4 count of $200/mm^3$ is of 38-40 months. Approximately 10% of the individuals rapidly evolve to AIDS 5 years after the HIV infection. Interestingly, as an exception, some patients remain stable, with a normal CD4 count, over lengthy periods of time. [5,10,11,12,14,16].

Clinical findings can predict the disease progression in HIV-positive patients. Oral candidiasis, hairy leukoplakia, unexplainable fever, diarrhea, and especially the development of pneumonia caused by *P.carinni* are factors independently associated to the progression of the infection to AIDS. Many laboratory tests have been used in order to predict the development of AIDS. Among HIV- positive patients, stratification based on the absolute number or the percentage of CD4+ helper T lymphocytes is still the best risk indicator for the disease evolution. Other studies that evaluate the development of AIDS include the total lymphocyte count lower than $4,000/mm^3$, hematocrit count lower than 40% and low percentage of CD4+ helper T lymphocytes [5,10,11,12,14,16].

Breakthroughs like the antiretroviral therapy and new prophylaxis methods have turned the course of the natural history of AIDS substantially, increasing the median life expectancy of patients. In the absence of therapy, the median life expectancy is approximately 9 months whereas with the adoption of a more aggressive treatment approach, this expectancy rises to 2-3 years. Before Elisa and Western Blot assays show positive results (3-12 weeks), the virus can be detected. PCR or bDNA (RNA viral load tests) usually reveal high viral loads, with a detection limit of 50 copies of HIV-1 RNA/ml. Acute symptoms generally last around 2-4 weeks, followed by clinical recovery and reduction of the plasmatic viremia, assumingly owing to the development of an immune response to the virus. A cytotoxic T lymphocyte response is related to the exponential reduction of HIV concentration in the peripheral blood which precedes the humoral response in many weeks. It is very likely that this initial burst of viremia is responsible for the distribution of the virus to the many organs, including the central nervous system, namely the brain and lymphoid tissues. The presence of symptomatic seroconversion and a prolonged disease state (over 14 days) seem to be correlated to a faster progression to AIDS. The virus biological properties may also play an important role in the HIV disease progression. Seroconversion usually occurs between 3-12 weeks after an established transmission event takes place. Almost all patients show seroconversion within three months after HIV transmission [5,10,11,12,14,16].

During the latency period after a primary infection, clinical laboratory exams usually show no alterations in results except for persistent generalized lymphadenopathy defined as the presence of unexplained enlarged lymph nodes in different areas (inguinal lymph nodes excluded) for a period of at least 3-6 months. At this moment the lymph tissue serves as a major reservoir for HIV, and the viral load in the peripheral blood is relatively low. Some studies on the natural history of HIV infection in male homosexuals show that the median CD4 count before the seroconversion is $1,000/mm^3$ with a decrease to a median of $670/mm^3$ one year after seroconversion. One year later, the rate of CD4+ T-lymphocyte decline is around 30-$90/mm^3$ [5,10,11,12,14,16].

The consequence of the progressive deterioration of the immune system that occur in most of HIV patients is the onset of clinically apparent diseases, namely the acquired immune deficiency syndrome (AIDS). At late stages, the architecture of lymph nodes is disrupted as follicular dendritic cells dissolve; thus, lymph nodes lose their function as viral reservoirs and give place to the systemic dissemination of the virus. The increase of the viral load in CD4+ T cells of the peripheral blood is associated with a progressive decline in CD4 count [5,10,11,12,14,16].

Cells are counted directly from the blood sample by laser flow cytometry. Through this method, monoclonal antibodies bind to the specific superficial structures on these cells which are stained with fluorophores. In some cases CD4+ T lymphocyte count can be expressed by the percentage of CD4 from the total amount of lymphocytes, in other words, a CD4 absolute count. In HIV negative individuals the normal value is around 40%; a CD4 percentage below 15% indicates a risk of severe infections. A persistent decrease in CD4+ T lymphocyte ratios can be observed among HIV-positive patients. However, many times this happens at a variable pace, and the count may remain stable for long periods of time [5,10,11,12,14,16,18].

The evolutive stages of the disease, according to the CD4+ T lymphocytes count, are classified as:

- **Acute infection or seroconversion (CD4 count between 1,000 and 500)**

This stage is generally asymptomatic. Symptoms like fever, adenopathy, pharyngitis, myalgia and transitory leucopenia occur within 2-6 weeks after the infection in 50% of the patients that develop the syndrome [5,6,7,12].

- **Early stage (CD4 count < 500)**

At this stage patients may present with lymphadenomegaly, dermatologic lesions and infections caused by *Varicella zoster*, *Herpes simplex* and *Epstein-Barr* viruses. The risk of death is lower than 5% within the period of 18-24 months after the acute infection stage [5,6,7,12].

- **Intermediate stage (CD4 count between 200 and 500)**

This is the phase in which bacterial opportunistic infections occur. This time the risk of death is 20-30% within the period of 18-24 months after the acute infection stage [5,6,7,12,18].

- **Late stage (CD4 between 50 and 200)**

Neoplasias (lymphoma and Kaposi's sarcoma), esophageal candidiasis and infections caused by *Pneumocystis carinii* and *Mycobacterium tuberculosis* frequently occur at this stage. The risk of death is between 50 and 70% within the period of 18-24 months after the acute infection stage [5,6,7,12,18].

- **Advanced stage (CD4 count < 50)**

Severe and disseminated infections, dementia, diarrhea, anorexia and an increase in the catabolism unrelated to neoplasias or the toxicity to medications usually occur [5,6,7,12,18].

16

4. GASTROINTESTINAL TRACT AND AIDS

It is estimated that 50 to 90% of the patients with AIDS have gastroenterological manifestations. Such events become more frequent according to the patient's immunodepression stage (CD4<500). The gastrointestinal tract (GIT) impairment may occur due to different etiopathogenies [12]:

- Opportunistic and non-opportunistic infections;
- neoplasias (Kaposi's sarcoma, lymphomas);
- HIV-related effects;
- medications.

A total of 72% of HIV-positive patients present gastrointestinal symptoms like diarrhea, dysphagia, anorexia and weight loss, nausea, vomiting and abdominal pain within the period of 36 months. However, all of the symptoms mentioned above, except for anorexia, are not always associated with the infectious or neoplastic pathology [12].

When it comes to AIDS, there is no pathognomonic feature of a specific agent. There are multiple agents in different organs, and not all syndromes can be associated with the HIV [12].

4.1 PANCREATIC MANIFESTATIONS

The pancreatic involvement in the course of AIDS may be AIDS-related or non-AIDS-related. As to AIDS-related pancreatic insufficiency, one can mention the following: opportunistic infections, neoplasias (Kaposi's sarcoma and lymphomas), intoxications caused by drugs used in the treatment and complications. Concerning non-AIDS-related events, the following examples are provided: alcohol-related acute or chronic pancreatitis, pancreatic adenocarcinoma, biliary pancreatitis or cholelithiasis, diabetes mellitus. Such events are found in the HIV negative population [5,6,7,9,12,18].

5. PANCREAS AND HIV

The pancreatic involvement in patients with AIDS is little described in the literature; however, it is often demonstrated in necropsy retrospective studies that the pancreatic involvement varies between 11-65%. Brivet *et al.* [21] revealed pancreatic involvement in 7 out of 13 necropsies;   Bricaine *et al.* [22] showed pancreatic involvement in 49 out of 113 necropsies; in Dowell *et al.* study, 52 pancreopathies out of 82 necropsies were identified; Bonacini [24] found 24% of AIDS-related pancreatic involvement among opportunistic infections and neoplasias (74/314); according to Chicarino et al. [25,26], three out of nine cases (33%), Klatt et al. mentioned 65 cases of pancreatic lesion in 565 necropsies (12%) [5,26] and Chehter et al. described 97 cases with pancreatic alterations in 177 necropsies (55%) [4,7,8].

Although little macroscopic alteration could be observed, when it came to the histopathological analysis of 109 necropsied patients, acinar atrophy was found in 60% of the cases, decrease in zymogen granules in acinar cytoplasm in 52%, nuclear abnormalities in 65%, pancreatic steatosis in 66% and focal necrosis in 17% of the cases. Acinar atrophy and steatosis suggest a nutritional problem [5]. In the ultrastructural exam a decrease in zymogene granules, enlargement and proliferation of the mitochondrial and endoplasmic reticulum, nuclear abnormalities and enlargement of lipid vesicles in the acinar cytoplasm could be observed [7,8,9].

Endoscopic retrograde pancreatographies reveal alterations in the pancreatic ducts in half of HIV-positive patients. Such alterations are similar to pancreatitis and are usually found in the AIDS-related sclerosing cholangitis. The abnormalities include dilatations, short stenosis of the pancreatic duct and side branch irregularities, which suggest chronic pancreatitis with possible increased serum amylases levels. The infection of the pancreas or the hepatobiliary tract by cytomegalovirus (CMV), microsporidia or mycobacteria may induce tubular irregularities and dilatation like in the sclerosing cholangitis. In pediatric patients non-specific alterations, like edema, inflammation, fibrosis, acinar secretion and macronesia were detected [7,8,9].

The pancreatic involvement is asymptomatic in 90% of the cases. The few laboratorial alterations that indicate the specific involvement of the organ make the diagnosis and a precise evaluation of the abnormalities very difficult to be accomplished. The major symptoms found were: fever (91%), weight loss (37%) and diarrhea (33%). The symptoms that suggest pancreatic involvement, like abdominal pain, were present in 15% of the cases without pancreatopathic features [7,8,9].

5.1 NON-AIDS-RELATED EVENTS

Acute and chronic pancreatitis, cholelithiasis, diabetes and adenocarcinoma are events that equally affect both HIV-positive individuals and the population in general. In a population-based retrospective study in the United States, rising rates of acute pancreatitis could be observed. Among 178 cases, a total of 5 etiologies were highlighted: biliary diseases (25%), alcohol (14%), idiopathic (22%), medication-induced (7%) and non-AIDS-related (12%) [5,6,7,8,9].

Alcoholic pancreatitis must be spotlighted owing to its influence not only on acute events but also on the aggravation of chronic cases. Although the incidence is the same as it is in the general population, the clinical course and prognosis are worse due to the nutritional condition and concomitant opportunistic infections [5,6,9,12].

There is a high incidence of vesicular lithiasis in patients with AIDS. Among 162 retrospectively analyzed HIV-positive patients, a total of 17% presented with gallbladder diseases and 14% with cholecystitis, a significantly higher rate than that in the HIV negative population [7,8,9].

Adenocarcinoma is not frequent in patients with AIDS [7,8,27] since these individuals are young and they are not part of the risk age group. Among the very few described cases, an unusual aggressive behavior was observed. It is little differentiated, histologically speaking, and its spread is fast with poor response to chemotherapy [7,8,27].

Concerning diabetes and AIDS, it is important to point out that the treatment requires a watchful monitoring of glycemia once there is not only a hepatic glycogen reserve, but also the association of opportunistic diseases with medications that induce hypoglycemia or hyperglycemia [7,8,27].

5.2 AIDS-RELATED EVENTS

The pancreatic involvement in AIDS can directly affect the gland or the organ without dysfunctional outcomes. It basically occurs due to 3 factors [7,8,9]:

1) Opportunistic infections;

2) medications used in the treatment of AIDS;

3) AIDS-related neoplasias.

The probable causes of pancreatopathies associated with AIDS are:

➤ Hyperamylasemia: It is a constant finding, and it is not always related to symptomatic pancreatic lesion. It occurs in 25% of ambulatory patients.

Sometimes amylasemia does not reflect a pancreatic involvement; it may represent an effect of renal insufficiency or macroamylasemia related to the polyclonal gammopathy of activated B lymphocytes [7,8,9].

In trying to make the diagnosis of pancreatic lesions in AIDS more accurate, other enzymes, such as trypsin and elastase-1, have been measured, and their levels are kept high throughout all stages of the disease [7,8,9]. Some studies revealed that there is an inverse relation between TCD4 lymphocyte count and the level of enzymes.

➤ Acute pancreatitis: In a multicentric case-control study, the rate of this event was 5%. A clinical similarity between HIV patients and the general population in relation to pancreatitis was observed. There were, however, besides a more complicated evolution and a higher mortality rate, differences concerning the high rates of drug-induced pancreatitis (18%) and the low incidence of biliary pancreatitis [7,8,9].
• In pediatric patients with AIDS, the rate of acute pancreatitis is in 17% of the cases [20].

➤ Chronic pancreatitis: No cases of chronic pancreatitis related to HIV, directly or indirectly, have been described [5,6,9].

5.3 INFECTIOUS AGENTS

The agents and the opportunistic infections that most affect the pancreas in order of frequency are: CMV, mycobacteriosis (TBC), toxoplasmosis, pneumocystosis, cryptococcosis, histoplasmosis, cryptosporidiosis, and rarely the ones mentioned below according the American literature. In a study with 109 necropsied patients in Brazil the following frequency was found: mycobacteria in 22% of the cases, toxoplasmosis in 13%, cytomegalovirus in 9%, *Pneumocistis carinii* in 9%, and HIV p24 antigen in cytoplasmic macrophage in 22% of the cases. The opportunistic infectious agents previously diagnosed in these patients were: TBC in 27% of the cases, toxoplasmosis in 17%, pneumonia caused by *Pneumocistis carinii in 49%,* infection caused by CMV in 13%, cryptococcosis in 5%, moniliasis in 4% and *Herpes zoster* in 3% of the cases [5,6,9,12].

5.4   VIRAL INFECTIONS

CMV is the virus more frequently found in HIV-positive patients, present in over 40% of the cases. Clinical manifestations only occur when CD4+ count is below 100 cells/mm³ [7,8,10,12].

At the final stage of the disease the CMV affects 20% of the patients, and it is mostly detected in the following areas: mouth, esophagus, stomach, small intestine, appendix and colon. In AIDS, although the CMV is the most frequent agent, there are only 7 acute pancreatitis cases caused by this virus described in the literature [28]. In necropsies of 109 patients with AIDS, the presence of the CMV was detected in 9% of the analyzed pancreases [5,6]. The pancreatic infection is asymptomatic, and diagnosis is made by necropsy with the presence of pathognomonic cell inclusions (owl's eye), demonstration of the antigen or the genomic material in the pancreatic tissue or the presence of the virus under microscopy analysis [5,6].

•   Herpes virus: In infected patients with CD4+ count above 100 cells/mm3, the clinical manifestations are similar to those in HIV negative patients. The viral dissemination through the body occurs in patients with low cell count, especially in the gastrointestinal tract, causing ulcers of the esophagus and intestine [7,8,10,12].

The diagnosis is made by means of the histopathological exam, which reveals typical cytopathic lesions with polynucleation, intranuclear inclusion bodies and nuclear ground glass appearance [5,6].

•   HIV: The direct action of the virus in the pancreas is still unknown. However, in a study with 109 necropsied patients with AIDS, HIV p24 antigen in cytoplasmic macrophage was found in 22% of the analyzed cases.
•   Other viruses: Some studies suggest the association of acute pancreatitis with viruses like *Epstein-Barr, Vaccinia,* Rubella, *Adenovirus.* No confirmation has been established yet [5,6,7,8].

5.5   BACTERIAL INFECTIONS

Among the pathogenic mechanisms, colonization originated from the small intestine or the biliary tract, along with hematogenous and lymphatic pathways, should be highlighted.

- *Mycobacterium tuberculosis*: Given the high virulence, it affects HIV carriers in the beginning of the infection, and one of its characteristics is the great number of extrapulmonary sites affected. Intra-abdominal tuberculosis usually involves the liver, spleen, bowel, mesenteric lymph nodes, and more rarely, the pancreas. Pancreatic tuberculosis may be either a manifestation of the dissemination or an isolated lesion. Some isolated cases of pancreatic abscess caused by tuberculosis have been reported, and necropsy studies reveal the presence of 22% of cases of pancreatic infection by *Mycobacterium tuberculosis* [5,6].
- Nontuberculous Mycobacteriosis: Leading to systemic disorders at the final stage of AIDS, this infection has as the most frequent agent the *Mycobacterium avium*, which is usually associated with other opportunistic diseases. The infection is asymptomatic, and it causes lymphocyte depletion, sharply reducing life expectancy of patients. Diagnosis is made by culture of aspirated material or by the histopathological exam of the pancreatic tissue through which aggregated macrophages, enlarged and foamy, stained by the Ziehl-Neelsen method with little inflammatory reaction can be observed. The early diagnosis of this agent is very important since the treatment helps increase the life expectancy of these patients [5,6,7,8,9].
- Leptospirosis: There is only one reported case of acute pancreatitis caused by leptospirosis in patients with AIDS [5,6,9].

5.6   FUNGAL INFECTIONS

These are the greatest causes of morbidity and mortality in patients with AIDS [5,6,7,8,9,10,12].

- Cryptococcosis: The incidence of this infection in HIV patients is between 6-30%. *Cryptococcus neoformans* is the disease causal airborne agent which spreads hematogenically in the immunosuppression. The gastrointestinal tract is rarely affected. However, whenever pancreatic impairment occurs, it is asymptomatic.

- Candidiasis: The most common etiologic agent is the *Candida albicans*, and it is the most frequent fungal infection in HIV patients. Causing mucosal manifestations, it compromises around 90% of AIDS patients at any stage of the disease, and 70% of the patients are affected in the gastrointestinal tract. Pancreatic candidiasis is extremely rare.

• Aspergillosis: Diagnosed by optical microscopy or tissue culture obtained by percutaneous aspiration or biopsy. Not common in AIDS events and pancreatic impairment is hardly found.

• Histoplasmosis: It is the most common endemic mycosis among AIDS patients. Contamination rate in endemic areas is around 75%. The gastrointestinal involvement is secondary and it spreads hematogenically. In HIV patients, histoplasmosis is related to T CD4 cell count, and it has been reported in 955 AIDS patients without specific manifestations. The pancreatic impairment in AIDS has been described in six necropsied cases and in one case of acute pancreatitis. Diagnosis is performed by isolation of the fungus from respiratory secretions, blood, bone marrow or by the analysis of the histoplasma polysaccharide antigen levels in the blood.

5.7 PROTOZOAN INFECTIONS

In AIDS, cases of pancreatic infections and acute pancreatitis caused by toxoplasmosis or cryptosporidia and cases of pancreatic lesion induced by pneumocystosis and microsporidia have been reported [5,6,7,8,9,10,12].

• Toxoplasmosis: It occurs in 10 to 15% of the HIV population. In a study with 80 necropsies of AIDS patients, a total of 13 cases (16%) of individuals with extracerebral toxoplasmosis were found: 15% in the cardiac muscle; 6% in the lungs; 5% in the pancreas; 6% in the GIT; 5% in the liver; 5% in the adrenals; 4% in the testicles. There are over 30 cases of pancreatic toxoplasmosis and fewer cases of acute toxoplasmic pancreatitis reported in the literature. Diagnosis is established by tissue culture, Giemsa staining patterns or by immunochemistry technique using cytoplasm specific antibodies.

• Pneumocystosis: Although pneumonia is highly prevalent in this population, extrapulmonary manifestations are not very common. Pancreatic impairment is a rare finding in necropsies.

• Cryptosporidiosis: Among all the species of cryptosporidia, the most pathogenic is the *Cryptosporidium parvum*. It is a prominent infection in HIV-positive and negative patients present in 8 to 37% of the former individuals and in 0.3 to 32% of the latter. It compromises the biliary tree, the pancreas, the gallbladder, the respiratory tract and especially in the GIT as the most common causal agent of AIDS-related diarrhea. In the biliary tract it leads to sclerosing cholangitis and acalculous cholecystitis. There are very few reports on pancreatic cryptosporidiosis or acute pancreatitis caused by this agent. The cryptosporidium was found in the pancreas of patients with intestinal cryptosporidiosis, more specifically located in the pancreatic ducts associated with squamous metaplasia of ductular epithelium with edema and periductal inflammatory infiltrate.

• Microsporidium: this is a rare pancreatic infection. The diagnosis is hard to be accomplished once the parasite is tiny in its size. Confirmation is made by electronic microscopy.

5.8 NEOPLASMS

Their incidence is inverse to the individual's immunocompetence. They are related to HIV infections in 12 to 40% of the cases, and the Kaposi sarcoma and lymphomas stand out with 95% of the cases. The GIT is compromised in 32% of the patients with AIDS-related neoplasia [5,6,7,8,9,10,12].

• Kaposi sarcoma: An opportunistic HIV-associated malignancy. The gastrointestinal impairment has been reported in 40 to 50% of the patients and it may occur without manifestations in different sites. The most affected gastrointestinal organ is the duodenum. Reported in more than 30 cases, the pancreatic impairment, a necropsy finding, is asymptomatic without clinical repercussion. The diagnosis is made by biopsy at which point the abnormal proliferation of vascular structures coated with enlarged endothelial cells and surrounded by fusiform cells can be observed in the histology. GTI impairment is a worse prognostic factor which decreases life expectancy.

• Lymphomas: The incidence has gradually increased since the beginning of the pandemia. Among the AIDS-related cases, Hodgkin and non-Hodgkin lymphomas, with an aggressive behavior in HIV patients, are highlighted.

6. AIDS TREATMENT – HAART

The High Active Antiretroviral Therapy (HAART), popularly known as "the cocktail", has been available since 1996 for the treatment of AIDS patients. It is a combination of drugs with different mechanisms of action classified as: Nucleoside Reverse Transcriptase Inhibitors (**NRTIs**), Nucleotide Reverse Transcriptase Inhibitors (**NtRTIs**), Non-Nucleoside Reverse Transcriptase Inhibitors (**NNRTIs**) and Protease Inhibitors (**PIs**). [10,11,12,14,19].

The antiretroviral therapy should start whenever CD4 count is lower than 350 or in patients with CD4 count between 350 and 500. However, the Panel on Clinical Practices for Treatment of HIV Infection has been established for patients with CD4 count higher than 500, with 50% in favor to the beginning of the antiretroviral therapy, and 50% in favor to the optional beginning of the therapy [10,11,12,14,19].

Many combinations of antiretroviral drugs are possible, based on clinical trials that establish the efficacy, adverse effects, interactions and facility in use. The recommended standard schema mappings are the following:

➢ **NRTI + NRTI + NNRTI**
➢ **NtRTI + NRTI**
➢ **NtRTI + NNRTI**
➢ **NRTI + NRTI + IP**
➢ **NRTI + IP + NRTI + IP**

The use of the combined therapy (HAART) increases the antiretroviral activity with elevated CD4+ T lymphocyte counts and reduction in plasma HIV RNA levels [10,11,12,14,19].

6.1 NNRTIs: NON-NUCLEOSIDE REVERSE TRANSCRIPTASE INHIBITORS

A class of drugs that binds directly and non-competitively to the enzyme at a site close to the nucleoside substrate binding site. The resulting complexes inhibit the active catalytic site of the viral reverse transcriptase enzyme, thus reducing nucleotide binding and the consequent polymerization. Contrary to NRTIs, NNRTIs do not require intracellular activation [10,11,12,14,19].

The main drugs in this class are:

NEVIRAPINE (NVP): It is able to suppress the viral load when used in the beginning of the infection. Some studies suggest that this drug may be effective in patients with high viral load or low CD4 count. In severe cases it may cause hepatotoxicity. It has a good lipid profile with favorable alterations in cholesterol and triacylglyceride levels [10,11,12,14,19].

DELAVIRDINE (DLV): An inhibitor of the cytochrome P450 and the CYP3A4 isoenzyme, it interacts with many other drugs. Although it is as effective as the other NNRTIs, it is rarely prescribed since, owing to its low half-life, a great number of tables is required. The most common adverse effect is the moderate to severe rash in up to 20% of the patients. Other common effects include fatigue, headaches, hepatotoxicity and nausea [10,11,12,14,19].

EFAVIRENZ (EFV): Combined with another retroviral, it acts as part of the post-exposition prophylaxis to prevent the HIV transmission. Possible effects in the central nervous system include morning dizziness, abnormal dreams, drowsiness and insomnia. It is not recommended during pregnancy. Hepatotoxicity is less frequent. Besides the collateral effects mentioned above, it may cause hyperlipidemia (hypercholesterolemia and hypertriglyceridemia) and an increase in transaminase and bilirubin levels [10,11,12,14,19].

6.2 PIs: PROTEASE INHIBITORS

These drugs act through a direct binding to a hydrophobic pouch close to the active site of the virus reverse transcriptase enzyme. This binding interrupts the HIV reverse transcriptase catalytic mechanism [10,11,12,14,19].

Below are listed the main drugs in this class:

RITONAVIR: It inhibits the enzymes that metabolize other protease-inhibiting drugs. This characteristic allows for reaching a plasma concentration level higher than in other set of drugs used together, thus increasing the clinical treatment efficiency. One of its collateral effects is hyperglycemia, which may cause type 1 diabetes [10,11,12,14,19].

ATAZANAVIR: Like other protease inhibitors, it is only used combined with other medications. It does not increase cholesterol and triacylglyceride levels, in contrast to other antiretroviral drugs of its class. It affects less the glicidic metabolism than the other protease inhibitors (less lipodystrophy and dyslipidemia) and it does not induce to insulin resistance. Collateral effects include jaundice and Gilbert's syndrome [10,11,12,14,19].

INDINAVIR: It prevents the development of drug-resistant HIV mutations, including resistance to other protease inhibitors. Nephrolithiasis is one of its collateral effects, affecting 5 to 25% of the patients; therefore, proper hydration during the treatment is recommended. Other collateral effects include hyperbilirubinemia (asymptomatic at times), hepatitis, mucocutaneous effects, alopecia and lip and dryness. Its greatest quality is the good CNS penetration when compared to other PIs [10,11,12,14,19].

AMPRENAVIR (APV): A non-peptidic competitive inhibitor of the HIV-protease. It blocks the ability of the viral protease to process viral precursor polyproteins necessary for the virus replication. Amprenavir is a powerful selective inhibitor of HIV-1 and 2 proteases. Its antiretroviral action undergoes synergetic interference when it is administered along with other antiretroviral drugs that act on the viral reverse protease, such as zidovudine, abacavir, didanosine, or other protease inhibitors, like saquinavir. Collateral effects include rashes in more than 30% of the cases and gastrointestinal effects [10,11,12,14,19].

SAQUINAVIR: A protease inhibitor with few collateral effects: mild gastrointestinal symptoms like nausea, diarrhea and abdominal discomfort [10,11,12,14,19].

NELFINAVIR (NFV): A protease inhibitor which may infrequently cause diarrhea, abdominal pain, hepatitis, nephrolithiasis, pancreatitis and leucopenia [10,11,12,14,19].

LOPINAVIR: Highly bound to plasma protein, it is used as a fixed-dose combination with another protease inhibitor, RITONAVIR. Adverse effects include nausea, diarrhea, dyslipidemia (much more severe than in other PIs) and lipodystrophy in 15% of the cases after 5 years of treatment [10,11,12,14,19].

6.3 NRTIs: NUCLEOSIDE REVERSE TRANSCRIPTASE INHIBITORS

With great effectiveness in zidovudine-intolerant individuals, this class of drugs acts as alternative substrates, namely false building blocks. They compete with physiological nucleosides from which they differ in a simple alteration of a sugar molecule [10,11,12,14,19]. Incorporation of nucleoside analogues inhibits DNA synthesis since phosphodiester bonds cannot be formed to stabilize the double-stranded structure. The nucleoside analogues are converted into active metabolites only after endocytosis, when they are phosphorylated to their triphosphate derivatives, interfering with the reverse transcriptase and becoming powerful inhibitors of the viral replication [10,11,12,14,19].

Most of the collateral effects are probably related to the mitochondrial toxicity. The mitochondrial function requires the presence of nucleosides. The metabolism of these cellular structures is disrupted by the incorporation of false nucleosides leading to mitochondrial degeneration. Nucleoside analogues are renally excreted, and hence there is no interference with other hepatic metabolized medications [10,11,12,14,19].

The main drugs in this class are:

ABACAVIR: It acts as a reverse transcriptase inhibitor which prevents viral replication by blocking the formation of HIV genetic material (RNA and DNA). A potent nucleoside analogue with good CNS penetration, abacavir has the hypersensitivity reaction (HSR) as its major adverse effect. It occurs in 93% of the patients in the first 6 weeks of treatment with flu-like symptoms, abdominal cramps, diarrhea and rash [10,11,12,14,19].

ZIDOVUDINE (AZT): This was the first-discovered antiretroviral drug which proved to be useful to extend life expectancy by reducing the frequency and severity of opportunistic diseases, partly though HIV replication suppression [14]. It is intracellularly phosphorylated to zidovudine monophosphate through cellular thymidine kinase; the monophosphate is further converted into diphosphate by cellular dimethyl kinase action and then it is converted into triphosphate through other cellular enzymes. Zidovudine triphosphate competes with the natural substrate, thymidine triphosphate, for incorporation into growing chains of viral DNA by retroviral reverse transcriptase (RNA-dependent DNA-polymerase). Once incorporated, zidovudine triphosphate prematurely interrupts the DNA-chain growth since the 3'-azido group prevents further 5'-3' phosphodiester linkages, therefore inhibiting the virus replication. Zidovudine affinity for the retrovirus reverse transcriptase is higher than the one for the human DNA-polymerase, and it allows the selective inhibition of the viral reproduction without blocking cellular replication. Anemia, neutropenia and leucopenia are possible side effects. Gastrointestinal issues like nausea and vomiting are short-term complaints [10,11,12,14,19].

ZALCITABINE (DDC): An HIV-replication inhibitor in low concentrations, it acts as a viral DNA chain terminator through its binding to the reverse transcriptase. As adverse effects, peripheral neuropathy, pancreatitis, macula-vesicular rash and stomatitis are included [10,11,12,14,19].

DIDADOSINE (DDI): This drug inhibits the viral replication. After the drug is modified inside the cell, it generates substrates that inhibit HIV reverse transcriptase and its replication as a result since it disrupts the virus' DNA synthesis. Gastrointestinal complaints are rather frequent. Pancreatitis occurrences are unusual, but as a secondary effect it may be fatal in some cases. Peripheral neuropathy and diarrhea are also reported adverse effects [10,11,12,14,19].

STAVUDINE (D4T): Stavudine inhibits HIV replication in human cell cultures. It is phosphorylated by cellular kinases to stavudine triphosphate, the active form of the drug, which inhibits HIV reverse transcriptase by competing with the natural substrate, thymidine triphosphate. It also inhibits the viral DNA synthesis by breaking the DNA chain owing to the absence of the 3'-hydroxyl group, which is necessary for the DNA elongation. Cellular DNA polymerase gamma is also sensitive to the inhibition by stavudine triphosphate whereas DNA polymerase alpha and beta are inhibited in concentrations, respectively, 4,000- and 40-fold higher than those necessary to inhibit HIV reverse transcriptase. Stavudine triphosphate sharply reduces DNA mitochondrial synthesis as well. In the beginning of the treatment it is better tolerated than AZT, causing fewer gastrointestinal side effects and reducing the risk of myelotoxicity (anemia). On the other hand, it increases the risk of lactic acidosis and hyperlactacidemia, lipodystrophy, pancreatitis, peripheral neuropathy, hepatotoxicity, as well as progressive muscular disease, with symptoms similar to the Guillain-Barré syndrome, in the long run [10,11,12,14,19].

LAMIVUDINE (3TC): A potent and selective inhibitor of HIV-1 and HIV-2 replication, lamivudine is intracellularly metabolized by the action of the active 5'-triphosphate, which has an intracellular half-life of 16-19 hours. Lamivudine 5'-triphosphate is a weak inhibitor in the RNA- and DNA-dependent activities of HIV reverse transcriptase. Its main mechanism of action is the inhibition of HIV reverse transcriptase, chain termination. It has been demonstrated that lamivudine acts additively and synergistically with other anti-HIV agents, zidovudine in particular, inhibiting replication of HIV in cell culture. It is also effective against Hepatitis B virus. The adverse effects that may occur due to its association with other drugs or the underlying pathologic state are: pancreatitis, peripheral neuropathy, malaise, fatigue, abdominal pain, paresthesia, exanthema, headache, nausea, vomiting, fever and diarrhea [10,11,12,14,19].

TENOFOVIR: Viread® is the trade name of the tenofovir disoproxil fumarate (a prodrug of tenofovir), which is a fumaric acid salt of bis-isopropoxycarbonyloxymethy ester derivative of tenofovir. The tenofovir disoproxil fumarate is converted to tenofovir, an acyclic nucleoside phosphonate (nucleotide) analog of adenosine 5-monophosphate. Tenofovir is active against HIV reverse transcriptase. Most common collateral effects include nausea, diarrhea, vomiting and flatulence [10,11,12,14,19].

7.   HAART VS. PANCREAS

Some pancreatitis cases are associated with the antiretroviral therapy. Many acute pancreatitis events, diagnosed by abdominal pain and an increase in the pancreatic amylase levels, have been attributed to the use of reverse transcriptase inhibitors like zidovudine, didanosine and stavudine in addition to the treatment with sulfamethoxazole-trimethoprim. As cumulative doses of such drugs are used, the risks are intensified. Didanosine and hydroxyurea may cause fatal pancreatitis. The use of pentamidine for the treatment of *P. carinii* in its both administration ways may result in acute necrotizing pancreatitis [7,9].

Some studies correlate exocrine pancreatic alterations with the malabsorption syndrome and diarrhea. The latter is, after all, a frequent morbidity cause among HIV-positive patients in the HAART era without further significant improvement over the course of time, due to its probable multifactorial origin. Pancreatic disorders appear as one of the causal factors of diarrhea. A study was performed with 35 HIV-infected patients and a set of 51 controls without gastroenterological diseases evaluating fecal elastase and fat by steatocrit test. In relation to elastase levels, control group showed normal values whereas 19 out of the 35 patients with AIDS (54%) had values significantly below normal in relation to the first group. An increase in the fecal excretion of elastase was observed in 25 out of 35 patients with AIDS (70%). Since opportunistic diseases and the administration of drugs exert no influence on elastase levels, the conclusion was that there is a reduction in exocrine pancreatic function with a decrease in elastase levels and an increase in malabsorption [29].

A similar result was found in a study conducted by Carroccio *et al.* It included 47 HIV-positive children, with no apparent pancreatic disease in relation to the 45 healthy individuals in the control set at the same age and of the same sex as in the infected group [29]. A total of 14 patients in the HIV group (30%) presented pancreatic function test with altered results: 7 with low elastase activity, 3 with chymotrypsin deficiency and 4 with lack of both enzymes. The values found in HIV patients were significantly lower than the ones found in the controls, and they were not associated with symptoms. A total of 12 children had steatorrhea and 4 of them showed increases in alpha-1 antitrypsin regardless of the disease stage, the antiretroviral therapy in use, nutritional and immunologic states or the presence of opportunistic diseases [29].

Concerning alterations in pancreatic enzyme levels and their causes, a total of 920 patients were evaluated in case-control study. Among this total, 334 individuals presented with at least one episode of alteration in at least 2 of the serum pancreatic enzymes and they were followed up over a long period of time. Among the 334 patients (36.3%), when compared with the control group, the only variables that showed a significant relation to the onset of occasional pancreatic disorders were: the long-term seropositivity, exposure to protease inhibitors, a more frequent immunodeficiency represented by the CD4+ T-lymphocyte count below 200, liver-biliary disease and hypertriglyceridemia. However, no relation between the administration and the length of the treatment with antiretrovirals was found [19].

From the 334 patients, 128 with prolonged laboratory alterations, with at least a three-fold higher increase in serum pancreatic enzymes over a period of 6 months or longer, were set aside. Association with clinical and ultrasonographic findings or signs of pancreatic involvement were detected in 32 patients. When compared with the other 206, the 128 individuals came up with the following aspects: they under continuous administration of didanosine, stavudine, pentamidine or cotrimoxazole, they were undergoing anti-tuberculosis therapy; they were alcohol abusers for over six months; they had opportunistic diseases with potential pancreatic involvement; they had chronic liver-biliary disease, exposure to protease inhibitors and hypertriglyceridemia; they had the combination of two or more corresponding factors. No differences were found among the 96 asymptomatics when compared with the 32 patients with clinical and ultrasonographic alterations [19].

Recurrence to enzymatic alterations occurred in over 70% of the patients, and in only 33.8% of the cases the antiretroviral therapy change was made necessary. Events of uncomplicated acute pancreatitis occurred in 7 out of the 26 symptomatic patients. With the administration of octreotide or gabexate in 59 out of the 128 cases for 2-4 weeks, there was an improvement in 71.2% of the cases, a higher rate of success of combination therapy over monotherapy. As a result, there was a decrease in number of recurrent diseases and a better tolerance to antiretrovirals [19].

These studies suggest the important role fecal elastase measurement plays in patients with diarrhea/weight loss or with steatorrhea, and in those whose antiretroviral treatment includes DDI so that pancreatic insufficiency may be detected in chronic diarrheic patients whenever other causes for diarrhea are excluded. When elastase levels are low, it is recommended that the antiretroviral medication be substituted for a treatment with orally administered pancreatic enzymes. Carroccio *et al.* [30] analyzed 24 HIV-infected patients with fat malabsorption. A total of 6 patients (25%) had low levels of elastase-1 and of fecal chymotrypsin and showed very high steatocrit values. The therapy with pancreatic enzymes was applied during 2-4 weeks, and in the 19 patients who concluded the study, steatocrit levels went back to the normal limit and their improvement was significantly higher than in those who did not undergo the treatment [19].

8.   JUSTIFICATION

The current known histological pattern of the pancreas in AIDS is from the pre-HAART era. Therefore, it is paramount to know the effects of the potent antiretroviral drugs (HAART) in the pancreas so that this pattern can be updated.

Have there been any changes since the introduction of the HAART? Histological findings of atrophy, steatosis, decrease in zymogen granules represent a pattern of protein-calorie malnutrition. Have there been any alterations in those findings? Do a higher life expectancy along with the immunological reconstruction have histological repercussion?

9.   OBJECTIVES

This study was conducted with 20 necropsies of AIDS patients under antiviral treatment at the SVOC-USP (Division of Postmortem Inspection at USP, São Paulo). The following aspects were analyzed:

• The populational sample and the comparison with other pancreatic samples obtained by necropsy from HIV patients who were not treated with antirevirals;

• the macro- and microscopic morphological aspects of the pancreas, comparing results found in the antiviral treated and untreated groups;

• the existence or non-existence of a histopathological pattern of the pancreas, characteristic in AIDS cases, after the treatment with antivirals;

• a possible secondary histopathological lesion after the treatment with antiretrovirals.

10.   PATIENTS AND METHODS

A prospective open sequential study was performed with 20 AIDS-diagnosed patients in use of HAART who were submitted to necropsy at the SVOC-USP (Division of Postmortem Inspection at USP, São Paulo) from June, 2006 to November, 2009. During that time, a set of 10 other cases were established as control group.

Exclusion criteria for the control group were the absence or suspicion of HIV-infection, diabetes mellitus, alcoholism, calculous cholecystopathy, infections or gastrointestinal complaints. Individuals who had died of cardiovascular causes were chosen. The 10 control-group cases are described below.

CONTROL GROUP (10 CASES) - (SVOC)

1.	**SVOC 7411/08: 67 y.o. female.**
•	Pancreas weight = 115 g
•	Cause of death: hemopericardium by aortic dissection
2.	**SVOC 7409/08: 39 y.o. female.**
•	Pancreas weight = 190 g
•	Cause of death: sudden death and systemic arterial hypertension (SAH)
3.	**SVOC 7619/08: 53 y.o. male.**
•	Pancreas weight = 145 g
•	Cause of death: pulmonary edema and hypertensive cardiopathy
4.	**SVOC 7626/08: 55 y.o. male.**
•	Pancreas weight = 148 g
•	Cause of death: acute myocardial infarction
5.	**SVOC 7631/08: 54 y.o. female**
•	Pancreas weight = 135 g
•	Cause of death: smoking and acute myocardial infarction
6.	**SVOC 7632/08: 45 y.o. male.**
•	Pancreas weight = 160 g
•	Cause of death: hemorrhagic cerebrovascular accident and hypertension
7.	**SVOC 7892/08: 58 y.o. male.**
•	Pancreas weight = 130 g
•	Cause of death: bilateral pulmonary thromboembolism
8.	**SVOC 7897/08: 65 y.o. female.**
•	Pancreas weight = 116 g
•	Cause of death: hemorrhagic cerebrovascular accident and systemic arterial hypertension
9.	**SVOC 7898/08: 48 y.o. male**
•	Pancreas weight = 155 g
•	Cause of death: aortic dissection and systemic arterial hypertension
10.	**SVOC 8130/08: 55 y.o. female.**
•	Pancreas weight = 150 g
•	Cause of death: pulmonary edema and hypertensive cardiopathy

This study was assisted by Dr Ana Maria Mader, MD, PhD, from the Pathology Department at ABC Medical School in Brazil. It was approved by the Research Ethics Committee from the referred institution under the number 141/2006, protocol CEP/FMABC. All patients were over 18 years old of age, diagnosed with AIDS, and they all made use of antiretroviral therapy.

20   CASES (2010) – HAART GROUP (SVOC)

1.	SVOC 10406/06: 44 y.o. male.
•	Pancreas weight = unknown
•	Cause of death: abscessed bronchopneumonia
2.	SVOC 11157/06: 31 y.o. male.
•	Pancreas weight = unknown
•	Cause of death: Hodgkin lymphoma
3.	SVOC 11163/06: 37 y.o. male.
•	Pancreas weight t = unknown
•	Cause of death: septicemia
4.	SVOC 11635/06: 35 y.o. male.
•	Pancreas weight = unknown
•	Cause of death: bronchopneumonia
5.	SVOC 11822/06: 31 y.o. male.
•	Pancreas weight = unknown
•	Cause of death: toxoplasmic meningoencephalitis
6.	SVOC 813/07: 46 y.o. male.
•	Pancreas weight = unknown
•	Cause of death: hepatocellular carcinoma
7.	SVOC 2394/07: 39 y.o. female.
•	Pancreas weight = unknown
•	Cause of death: toxoplasmic necrotizing encephalitis
8.	SVOC 9406/07: 49 y.o. male.
•	Pancreas weight = unknown
•	Cause of death: bronchopneumonia
9.	SVOC 9904/07: 31 y.o. male.
•	Pancreas weight = 110 g
•	Cause of death: disseminated atypical mycobacteriosis
10.	SVOC 6885/08: 35 y.o. male.
•	Pancreas weight = 68 g

•	Cause of death: bronchopneumonia
11.	**SVOC 7231/08: 46 y.o. male.**
•	Pancreas weight = 150 g
•	Cause of death: ischemic-hypertensive cardiopathy
12.	**SVOC7243/08: 25 y.o. male.**
•	Pancreas weight = 66 g
•	Cause of death: toxoplasmic pericarditis
13.	**SVOC 8869/08: 46 y.o. male.**
•	Pancreas weight = 68 g
•	Cause of death: bronchopneumonia
14.	**SVOC 9371/08: 39 y.o. male.**
•	Pancreas weight = 110 g
•	Cause of death: disseminated atypical mycobacteriosis
15.	**SVOC 10055/08: 51 y.o. male.**
•	Pancreas weight = 88 g
•	Cause of death: septicemia
16.	**SVOC 12435/08: 41 y.o. male.**
•	Pancreas weight = 120 g
•	Cause of death: disseminated cryptococcosis
17.	**SVOC 479/09: 28 y.o. female.**
•	Pancreas weight = 60 g
•	Cause of death: toxoplasmic necrotizing encephalitis
18.	**SVOC 1932/09: 60 y.o. male.**
•	Pancreas weight = 106 g
•	Cause of death: bronchopneumonia
19.	**SVOC 2028/09: 49 y.o. male.**
•	Pancreas weight = 154 g
•	Cause of death: bronchopneumonia
20.	**SVOC 5639/09: 44 y.o. female.**
•	Pancreas weight = 85 g
•	Cause of death: bilateral bronchopneumonia

Characterization of HIV Group

All the information was not only obtained from the medical record of each necropsied patient, but also from the data supplied by interviews with family members.

Analyzed topics:

➢   Age
➢   Sex
➢   Race
➢   BMI (body mass index = weight/height^2)
➢   Marital status
➢   I.V. drug use
➢   Alcoholism

Most consumed alcoholic beverages:

➢   Sugar cane liquor (*cachaça*)
➢   Beer

Smoking:

➢   A total of 15 patients were smokers.

HIV treatment:

➢   Antiretrovirals.

Medications employed for the treatment:

NRTIs	PIs	NNRTIs
ABACAVIR	RITONAVIR	NEVIRAPINE (NVP)
ZIDOVUDINE (AZT)	ATAZANAVIR	DELAVIRDINE (DLV)
ZALCITABINE (DDC)	INDINAVIR	EFAVIRENZ (EFV)
DIDANOSINE (DDI)	AMPRENAVIR (APV)	
STAVUDINE (D4T)	SAQUINAVIR	
LAMIVUDINE (3TC)	NELFINAVIR (NFV)	
TENOFOVIR	LOPINAVIR	

Treatment time:

➢ Minimum of 1 year and maximum of 20 years, with an average of 3 years of treatment.

HIV treatment locations:

➢ Santo Amaro Community Health Center, Freguesia do Ó Community Health Center, Emilio Ribas Hospital.

Death locations:

➢ Mandaqui Hospital, Jabaquara Hospital, Regional Sul Hospital, Campo Limpo Hospital, Emilio Ribas Hospital, Nossa Senhora da Penha Hospital, Vila Nova Cachoerinha General Hospital, Guaianases General Hospital, Campo Limpo Hospital Emergency Room, Pirituba Hospital Emergency Room and home.

Cause of death: abscessed bronchopneumonia, Hodgkin lymphoma, septicemia, toxoplasmic meningoencephalitis, hepatocellular carcinoma, toxoplasmic necrotizing encephalitis, disseminated atypical mycobacteriosis, hypertensive and ischemic cardiopathy, toxoplasmic pericarditis and disseminated cryptococcosis.

Other AIDS-related previous diseases:

➢ Previous opportunistic infections
➢ Neoplasias

Considered clinical manifestations:

➢ Fever
➢ Weight loss
➢ Acute or chronic diarrhea

Symptoms related to pancreatic impairment:

➢ Abdominal pain (localized or diffuse, epigastric or non-epigastric, with or without radiation)
➢ Diabetes mellitus
➢ Steatorrhea

Pathologic anatomy:

All readings of slides, necropsies in HIV-positive subjects and pathology reports were performed by one single experienced pathologist at SVOC/USP.

Macroscopy:

During necropsy examination, after the removal of the viscera, the pancreas was resected, weighed in grams, and the presence of lesions like hemorrhage, necrosis, fibrosis or tumor was reported.

The analysis proceeded to:

➢ Sequential transversal sectioning of the pancreas.
➢ Removal of significant samples from the head, body and tail (one from each region), separately designated.
➢ Fixation of the samples in 10% buffered formalin.

Preparation of slides for microscopy:

The obtained pancreatic fragments were routinely processed for further histological analysis. They were then dehydrated in graded alcohols and cleared in xylene for paraffin immersion. The paraffin blocks were submitted to histological sections of 4 μm, placed on slides and stained by standard hematoxylin-eosin technique (HE). Finally, the slides were mounted on glass coverslips coated with balsam.

Optical microscopy procedure:

The histopathological analysis was performed using a Nikon binocular microscope with five achromatic objective lenses. The analysis included: acinar cells and lumen, interlobular and intralobular pancreatic ducts (dilation and protein plugs in the lumina), abnormalities in the stroma (presence or absence of inflammatory infiltrate, edema, hemorrhage, fibrosis and steatosis) and islets of Langerhans. The presence or absence of lesions like necrosis, granulomas and neoplasias were also evaluated.

Semi-quantitative analysis:

The alterations found were quantified by semi-quantitative method with the following rating scale:

➤   0 (zero) = absent
➤   1 (one) = mild
➤   2 (two) = moderate
➤   3 (three) = severe

CHARACTERIZATION OF PANCREATITIS AND FOCI OF LYMPHOMONONUCLEAR INFLAMMATORY INFILTRATE:

Pancreatitis was defined according to the criteria established by the Atlanta classification (1992) [32,33].

➤   It is characterized by a necrotic and inflammatory process with a sharp onset whose morphologic alterations range from interstitial edema and minimum histological alterations to large confluent areas of necrosis and hemorrhage. At first the center of the lesion is located around the steatonecrosis perilobular, extending to bordering vessels, acinar cells and duct cells.

➤   The focus of lymphomononuclear inflammatory infiltrate was characterized as an aggregate of lymphocytes and/or plasma cells, unifocal or multifocal in the stroma, as a result of the inflammatory process of the pancreas. Its progression may result in scarring process and loss of exocrine and endocrine pancreatic functions.

Histochemistry:

In order to analyze fibrosis, besides the standard staining by HE, Masson's trichrome histochemical technique was also carried out as described below:

•   First sections were deparaffinized and hydrated in distilled water;

- next they were fixated in Bouin's solution for one hour, at a temperature of 56°C, and then rinsed in tap and distilled water;
- after that they were slightly stained in hematoxylin for 2-5 seconds and rinsed in tap and distilled water;
- next they were stained in Biebrich scarlet-acid fuchsin solution for 5-10 seconds and again they were washed in tap and distilled water;
- sections were stained in differentiation solution for 3-5 seconds and rinsed in tap and distilled water;
- they were then stained in aniline blue for 10 seconds and rinsed in distilled water;
- the samples were immersed in acetic water solution (1%) and rapidly rinsed;
- after that they were bathed in 96% alcohol, absolute alcohol and xylol;
- finally they were mounted on balsam-coated coverslips.

Periodic Acid-Schiff stain (PAS):

- Sections were deparaffinized, hydrated and washed in distilled water;
- then they were oxidized in periodic acid for 5-10 minutes;
- next they were immersed in distilled water for 10 minutes;
- the sections were stained in Schiff's reagent for 15 minutes;
- right after that they were washed in tap water until a bright shade of pink was achieved;
- they were then placed in Carazzi's hematoxylin for 3 minutes and rinsed in tap water for 5 minutes;
- the samples were dehydrated in 95% alcohols, absolute alcohols, and had two successive passages in xylol;
- finally they were mounted on balsam-coated coverslips [31,34].

Fite-Faraco stain:

- Sections were deparaffinized and hydrated in distilled water;
- next they were immersed in fuchsin solution for 30 minutes and then rinsed in tap water;
- the samples were briefly immersed in a differentiation solution and then rinsed in tap water for 5 minutes;
- after that they were counterstained with methylene blue for one minute and rinsed in tap water;
- samples were finally immersed in xylol before balsam-coated slides were mounted [31,34].

Immunohistochemistry:

The immunohistochemistry analysis was performed for the monoclonal mouse anti-cytomegalovirus antibody (CMV- clone MO854 - Dako) and the monoclonal mouse anti-pneumocystis carinii antibody (PMC - clone MOB 091 -05 Dako) in histological sections of 4 µm. They were mounted on slides previously silanized and stored in the lab oven (60°C) for 24 hours according to the following reaction protocol:

- Sections were deparaffinized with hot xylol (60°C) for 15 minutes and then at room temperature for 15 minutes;
- next, they were hydrated in decreasing concentrations of alcohol (100, 95, 80 and 70% respectively for 30 seconds each) followed by washes in tap and distilled water;
- after that, the sections were heated in a pressure cooker, for both antibodies, for 5 minutes after boiling in citrate buffer;
- endogenous peroxidase was blocked with 6% hydrogen peroxide diluted with methanol (volume by volume), 6 immersions of 5 minutes each;
- the slides were rinsed in tap water, distilled water and phosphate buffered saline solution (PBS 10mM, pH 7.4);
- they were overnightly incubated with primary antibodies of CMV (1:50) and Pc (1:250) in 1% BSA (bovine serum albumin) at 4°C in a humid chamber;
- the sections were then washed in PBS;
- the next step was to incubate the slides with biotinylated secondary antibodies (LSAB-plus) from the LSAB 2 kit/HRP, Rabbit/Mouse –Dako at 37 °C for 20 minutes;
- the sections were again washed in PBS;
- the following stage was to incubate the slides with the streptavidin-biotin-peroxidase complex at 37 °C for 20 minutes;
- the reaction was revealed by using the following chromogenic substrate: 60 mg of diaminobenzidine, 1mL of 20-volume hydrogen peroxide,   100 mL of PBS and 1 mL of dimethyl sulfoxide at   37 °C for 5 minutes, light protected; microscopic analysis showed the formation of a dark brown precipitate on the positive control slides as the final product of the reaction;
- after that, the sections were counterstained with Harris hematoxylin for 1 minute, and then immersed in ammonia water; wash in tap and distilled water followed the process;
- next, they were dehydrated in increasing concentrations of ethyl alcohol (70, 80, 95 and 100%);

• the sections were finally immersed in xylol and mounted on balsam for optical microscope analysis.

The HAART group (2010), composed of 20 pancreatic samples, was compared with the pre-HAART group (1995), with 109 samples, so that alterations resulted from the use of medications during this period could be identified.

11. STATISTICAL ANALYSIS

Initially all variables were descriptively analyzed. As to quantitative variables, this analysis was made by observing the maximum and minimum values and by calculating the means, standard deviation and medians. Regarding qualitative variables, absolute and relative frequencies were calculated.

The Student's t-test was use to compare the means between two groups.

The Chi-Square test or the Fisher's exact test whenever expected frequencies were lower than 5, was applied to evaluate the homogeneity between the proportions. In all tests, the p value was considered significant when ≤ 0.05.

The Mann-Whitney test was used to verify the differences in the distribution among the 20 cases (HAART group) and the 10 cases (control group) (p value < 5).

12. RESULTS

Table A: Mann-Whitney test to verify the differences in the distribution among the 20 cases in the HAART group and the cases in the control group.

. Variables	p
Decreased ZG levels	<0.001
Displasia	**0.480**
Atrophy	<0.001
Steatosis	0.001
Infflamation	0.023
Enlarged islets	**0.002**
Islet dysplasia	**0.309**
Pancreas weight	**0.003**

As seen in the table above, there were statistically significant differences for all variables in relation to the HAART group (20 cases), except for dysplasia (p=0.480) and dysplasic islets (p=0.309).

Values of pancreas weight in the HAART group (20 cases) were higher when compared with the control group.

The tables below show the comparisons between these two groups (non-HAART and HAART groups). All data were collected in the years 1995 (n=109; 84.5%) and 2010 (n=20; 15.5%).

Table 1. AIDS: anthropometric data and pancreas parameters in the years 1995 (n=109) and 2010 (n=20).

Age variable (in years)	Category	Year 1995 (n=109)	2010 (n=20)	P
		37.39 ± 10.09	40.35 ± 8.87	$0.223^{(1)}$
Pancreas weight (in grams)		**138.80 ± 33.10**	98.75 ± 31.92	$< 0.001^{(1)}$
BMI		20.68 ± 2.72	20.70 ± 3.28	$0.981^{(1)}$
Sex	Male	80 (73.4%)	17 (85.0%)	$0.400^{(2)}$
	Female	29 (26.9%)	3 (15.0%)	
	White	66 (60.6%)	13 (65.0%)	
Ethnicity	Mixed-races	29 (26.6%)	4 (20.0%)	$0.818^{(3)}$
	Black	14 (12.8%)	3 (15.0%)	
	Single	70 (64.2%)	16 (80.0%)	
Marital status	Married	26 (23.9%)	2 (10.0%)	$0.493^{(2)}$
	Widowed	9 (8.3%)	1 (5.0%)	
	Divorced	4 (3.7%)	1 (5.0%)	

(1) Descriptive level of probability of the Fisher's exact test
(2) Descriptive level of probability of the chi-square test

According to the table above, both groups differ in relation to pancreas weights. The 1995 group had values significantly higher than the 2010 group.

Table 2. General clinical manifestations, alcoholism, smoking, pancreatic manifestations and medications in use during AIDS treatment in the years 1995 (n=109) and 2010 (n=20)

	Year				
	1995 (n=109)		**2010 (n=20)**		
Signs and symptoms	n	%	n	%	p
Fever	**99**	**90.8**	4	20.0	$< 0.001^{(1)}$
Weight loss	40	36.7	12	60.0	$0.051^{(2)}$
Diarrhea	36	33.0	8	40.0	$0.545^{(2)}$
Abdominal pain	11	10.1	**6**	**30.0**	$0.027^{(1)}$
Alcoholism	23	21.1	**18**	**90.0**	$< 0.001^{(2)}$
Smoking	29	26.6	**15**	**75.0**	$< 0.001^{(2)}$
Diabetes	0	0.0	**2**	**10.0**	$0.023^{(1)}$
NRTI (mean in 3 years)	0	0.0	**19**	**95.0**	$< 0.001^{(1)}$
AZT (mean in 3 years)	39	35.8	**18**	**90.0**	$< 0.001^{(2)}$
NNRTI (mean in 3 years)	0	0.0	**2**	**10.0**	$0.023^{(1)}$
PI (mean in 3 years)	0	0.0	**3**	**15.0**	$0.003^{(1)}$

(1) Descriptive level of probability of the Fisher's exact test
(2) Descriptive level of probability of the chi-square test

According to the table above, both groups differ in relation to the presence of fever, abdominal pain, diabetes, alcoholism, NRTI, AZT, smoking habit, NNRTI and PI. Higher rates of fever can be observed in the 1995 group when compared with the 2010 group. As to the other variables, higher rates are found in the 2010 group.

Table 3A. AIDS: semi-quantitative microscopic aspects of acinar components, the pancreatic stroma; histological aspects of acini, ducts and pancreatic lesions, classified in levels, in the years 1995 (n=109) and 2010 (n=20).

Variable	Year	Absent	Mild	Moderate	Severe	p*
			Level			
Decreased ZG level	1995	52 (47.7%)	52 (47.7%)	5 (4.6%)	0 (0.0%)	< 0.001
	2010	1 (5.0%)	9 (45.0%)	6 (30.0%)	4 (20.0%)	
Displasia-like	1995	35 (32.1%)	48 (44.0%)	19 (17.4%)	7 (6.4%)	< 0.001
	2010	19 (95.0%)	0 (0.0%)	0 (0.0%)	1 (5.0%)	
Atrophy	1995	44 (40.4%)	45 (41.3%)	17 (15.6%)	3 (2.8%)	0.017
	2010	2 (10,0%)	13 (65,0%)	3 (15,0%)	2 (10,0%)	
Steatosis	1995	36 (3.0%)	43 (39.5%)	23 (21.1%)	7 (6.4%)	0.689
	2010	7 (35.0%)	7 (35.0%)	6 (30.0%)	0 (0.0%)	
Inflammation	1995	59 (54.1%)	39 (35.8%)	7 (6.4%)	4 (3.7%)	0.673
	2010	12 (60.0%)	5 (25.0%)	2 (10.0%)	1 (5.0%)	
Hemorrhage	1995	78 (71.6%)	26 (23.9%)	4 (3.7%)	1 (0.9%)	0.921
	2010	14 (70.0%)	5 (25.0%)	1 (5.0%)	0 (0.0%)	
Fibrosis	1995	67 (61.5%)	22 (20.2%)	16 (14.7%)	4 (3.7%)	0.173
	2010	8 (40.0%)	6 (30.0%)	6 (30.0%)	0 (0.0%)	

(*) Descriptive level of probability of the Fisher's exact test

Table 3B. AIDS: semi-quantitative microscopic aspects of acinar components, the pancreatic stroma; histological aspects of acini, ducts and pancreatic lesions, classified in levels, in the years 1995 (n=109) and 2010 (n=20).

Variable	Year	Level Absent	Mild	Moderate	Severe	p*
Plugs	1995	107 (98.2%)	2 (1.8%)	0 (0.0%)	0 (0.0%)	0.026
	2010	17 (85.0%)	3 (15.0%)	0 (0.0%)	0 (0.0%)	
Necrosis	1995	91 (83.5%)	18 (16.5%)	0 (0.0%)	0 (0.0%)	0.057
	2010	18 (90.0%)	1 (5.0%)	1 (5.0%)	0 (0.0%)	
Apoptosis	1995	109 (100.0%)	0 (0.0%)	0 (0.0%)	0 (0.0%)	
	2010	4 (20.0%)	8 (40.0%)	7 (35.0%)	1 (5.0%)	< 0.001
Enlarged	1995	109 (100.0%)	0 (0.0%)	0 (0.0%)	0 (0.0%)	
Islets	2010	8 (40.0%)	9 (45.0%)	3 (15.0%)	0 (0.0%)	< 0.001
Islests with	1995	109 (100.0%)	0 (0.0%)	0 (0.0%)	0 (0.0%)	0.023
dysplasia-like alterations	2010	18 (90.0%)	2 (10.0%)	0 (0.0%)	0 (0.0%)	

(*) Descriptive level of probability of the Fisher's exact test

According to what has been displayed in tables 3A and 3B, the following points should be considered:

1) The groups differ in relation to decrease in levels of ZG (zymogen granules): the 2010 group shows lower rates of absent and mild cases and higher rates of moderate to severe cases when compared with the 1995 group;

2) the groups differ in relation to dysplasia-like alterations: the 2010 group shows higher rates of absent cases and lower rates of the other cases when compared with the 1995 group;

3) the groups differ in relation to atrophy: the 2010 group shows higher rates of mild cases and lower rates of the other cases when compared with the 1995 group;

4) the groups differ in relation to secretion retention: the 2010 group shows higher rates of mild cases and lower rates of the other cases when compared with the 1995 group;

5) the groups differ in relation to apoptosis: the 2010 group shows higher rates of mild, moderate and severe cases and lower rates of absent cases when compared with the 1995 group;

6) the groups differ in relation to enlarged islets: the 2010 group shows higher rates of mild and moderate cases and lower rates of absent cases when compared with the 1995 group;

7) the groups differed in relation to islets with dysplasia-like alterations: the 2010 group shows higher rates of mild cases and lower rates of absent cases when compared with the 1995 group.

Table 4: Acute pancreatitis, foci of lymphomononuclear inflammatory infiltrate and opportunistic infections detected at necropsy in the years 1995 (n=109) and 2010 (n=20).

	Year				
	1995 (n=109)		**2010 (n=20)**		
Presence of characteristics	n	%	n	%	p*
Acute pancreatitis	10	9.2	0	0.0	0.360
Foci of lymphomononuclear inflammatory infiltrate	9	8.3	**12**	**60.0**	<0.001
Microbacteria	21	19.3	2	10.0	0.525
Fungi	4	3.7	1	5.0	0.576
Bacteria	10	9.2	0	0.0	0.360
Protozoa	16	14.7	0	0.0	0.131

(*) Descriptive level of probability of the Fisher's exact test

According to the table above, both groups differ in relation to the presence of foci of lymphomononuclear inflammatory infiltrate: the 1995 group shows lower rates of cases when compared with the 2010 group.

Table 5. AIDS and pancreas: immunohistochemical reactions for the characterization of infectious agents in the years 1995 (n=109) e 2010 (n=20).

Variables	Year				
	1995 (n=109)		2010 (n=20)		
	n	%	n	%	P*
CMV	10	9.2	0	0.0	0.360
Pc	15	13.8	0	0.0	0.125

(*) Descriptive level of probability of the Fisher's exact test
CMV= cytomegalovirus
Pc= Pneumocystis carinii

According to the table above, the groups do not show significant differences in relation to those variables.

12.1 PANCREATIC HISTOLOGICAL ANALYSIS IN THE HAART ERA

➢ The following was evaluated in acinar cells:

Zymogen granules in the acinar cytoplasm (**Figures 4 and 5**).

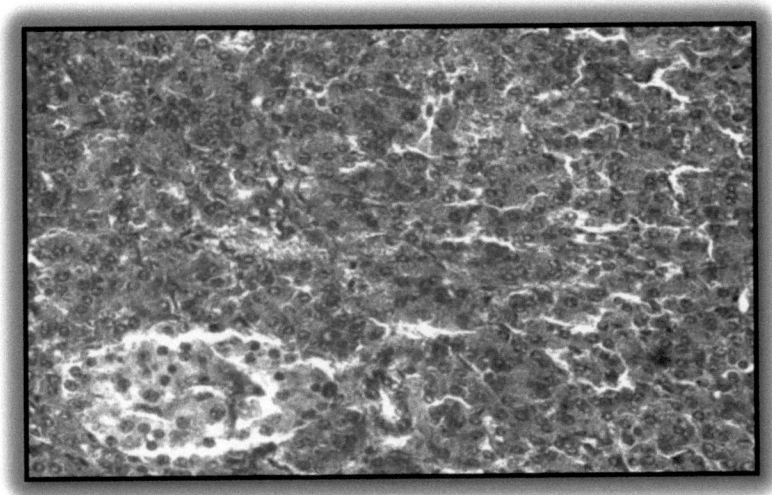

Figure 4 (HE 40x): Control group. Preserved amount of zymogen granules in the cytoplasm of acinar cells

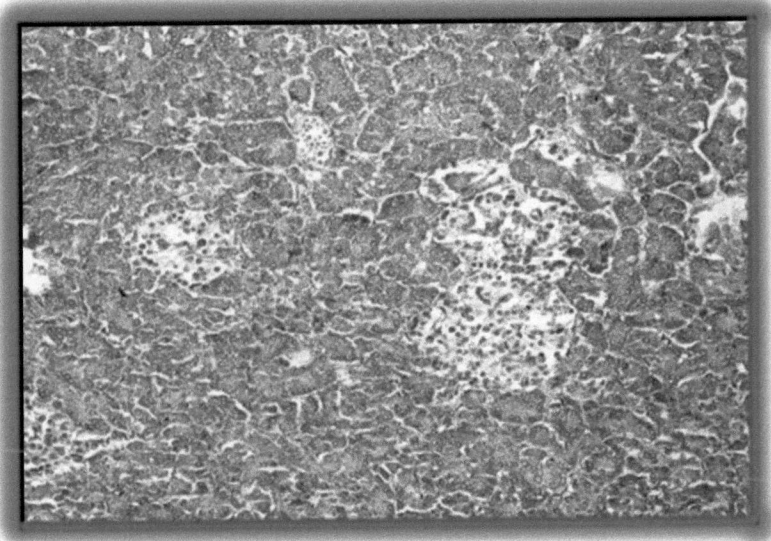

Figure 5 (HE 20x): Case 4. Depletion of zymogen granules in acinar cells characterized by the pale eosinophilic staining.

➤ The presence or absence of dysplasia-like lesions in the acinar cell nucleus. This aspect was taken into consideration whenever there was an increase in the nuclear volume and when the nucleus was hyperchromatic, with dense chromatin, irregular and thickened contours (**Figure 6**).

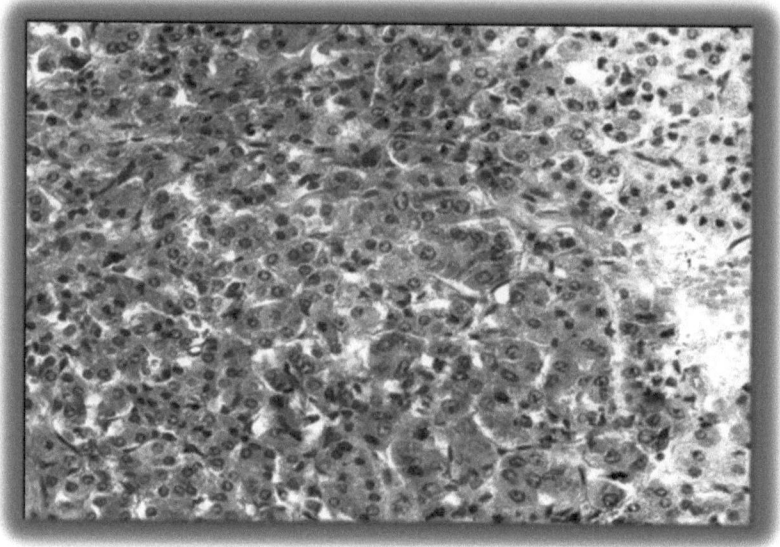

Figure 6 (HE 40x): Case 2. Dysplasia like alterations in acinar cell nuclei such as karyomegaly and evident nucleolus.

➤ The presence or absence of apoptosis. Unequivocally identified cells according to the Kerr criteria [31] were taken into consideration, namely, those cells with eosinophilic cytoplasm and chromatin condensation, and the presence of nuclear fragmentation without inflammatory reaction around.

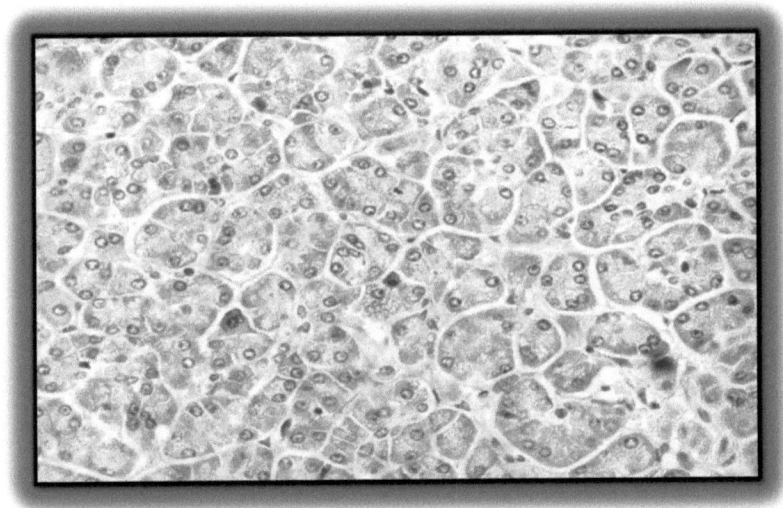

Figure 7 (PAS 40x): Case 2. Presence of apoptotic bodies in the pancreatic acini.

➢ Acinar cell size (**Figures 8 and 9**).

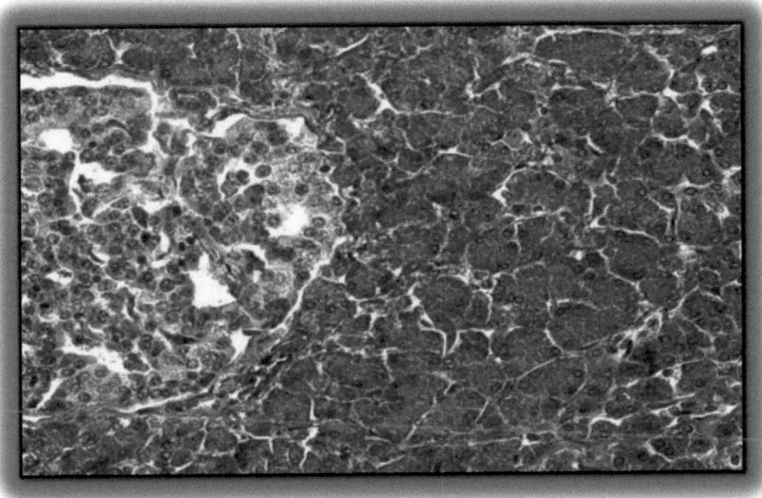

Figure 8 (HE 20x): Control group. Acinar cells of adequate sizes.

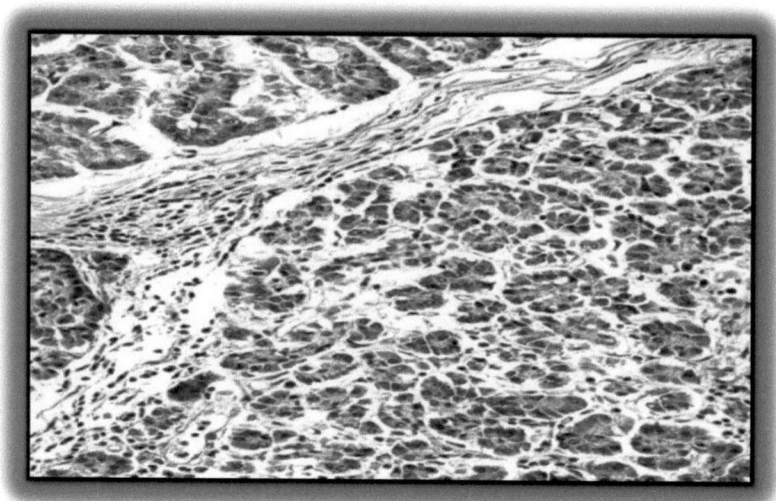

Figure 9 (HE 20x): Case 12. Presence of atrophy of the pancreatic acini.

➢ Analysis of acinar lumen (**Figure 10**).

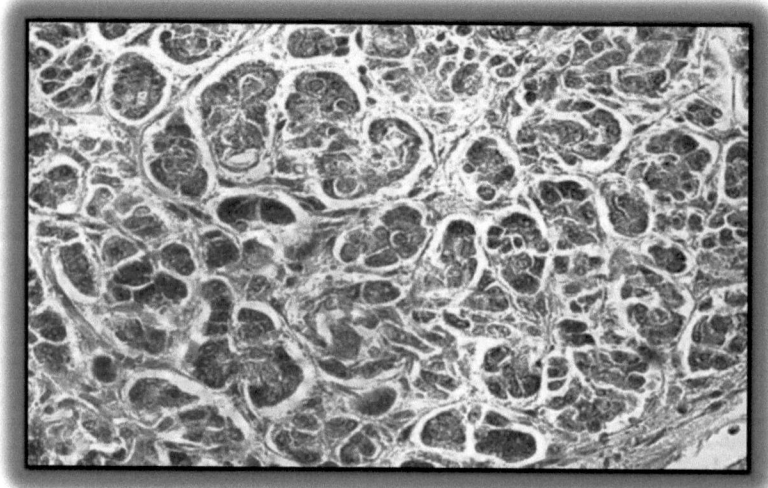

Figure 10 (PAS 40x): Case 9. Presence of acinar lumen dilation caused by secretion plugs.

➢ Evaluation of pancreatic ducts (protein plugs and calcifications) (**Figure 11**).

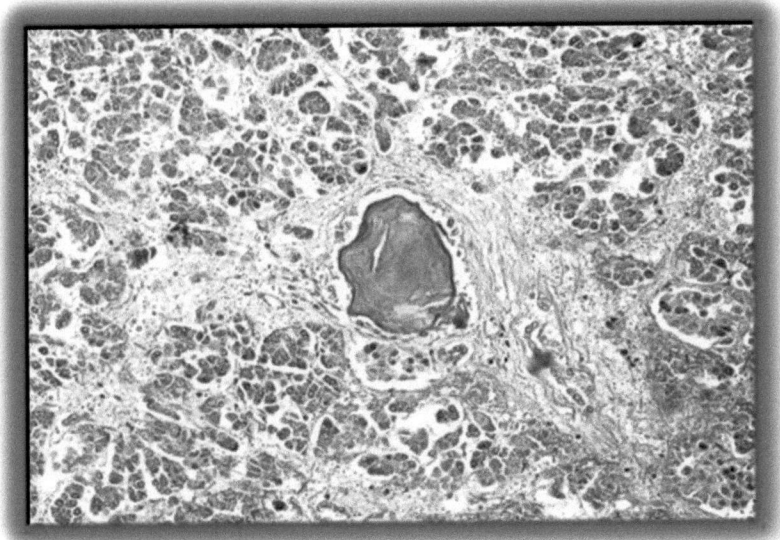

Figure 11 (HE 10x): Case 18: Presence of protein plugs in ducts.

➢ The following was evaluated in the Langerhans islets:

Alterations in the number and volume of the islets as well as dysplasia-like alterations in the nuclei of these cells (**Figures 12, 13A and 13B**).

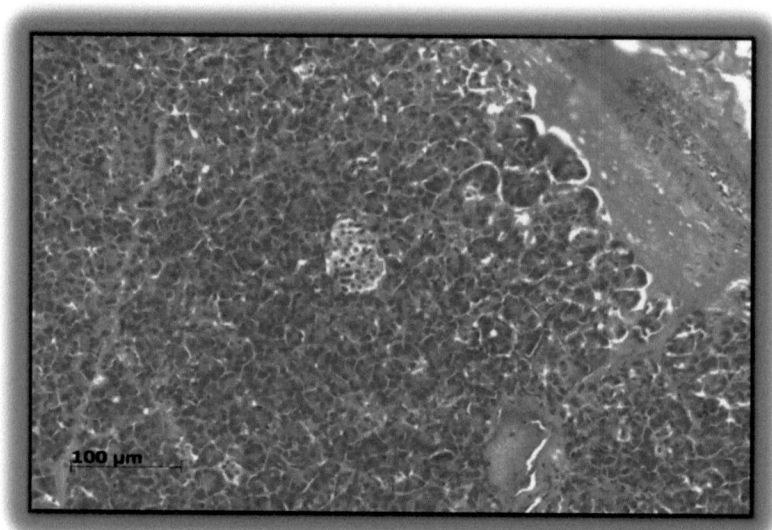

Figure 12 (HE 20x): Control group. Langerhans islets in their preserved size.

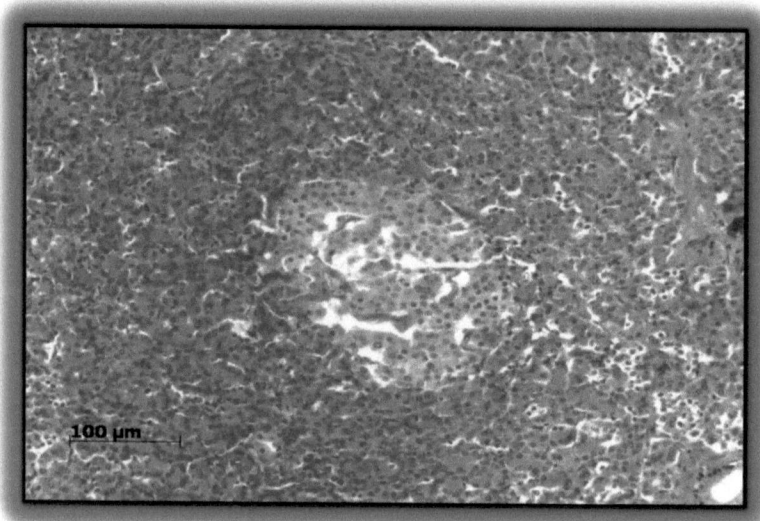

Figure 13A (HE 20x): Case 12. Presence of enlarged Langerhans islet.

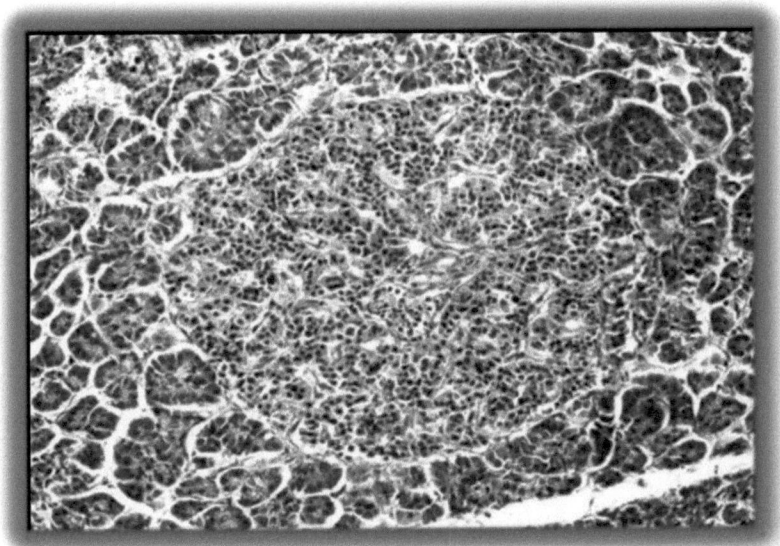

Figure 13B (HE 20x): Case 12. Presence of enlarged Langerhans islet.

➢ Steatosis and inflammatory infiltrate were evaluated in the stroma.

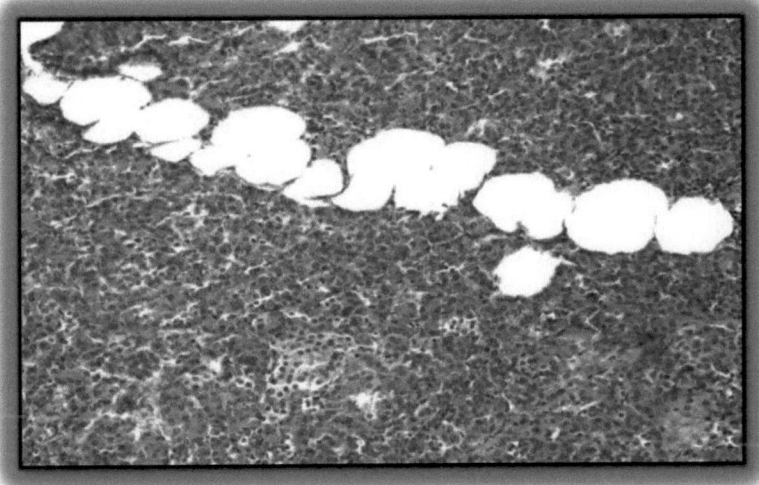

Figure 14 (HE 20x): Case 20. Presence of adipocytes characterized by vacuolar spaces between pancreatic acini (steatosis).

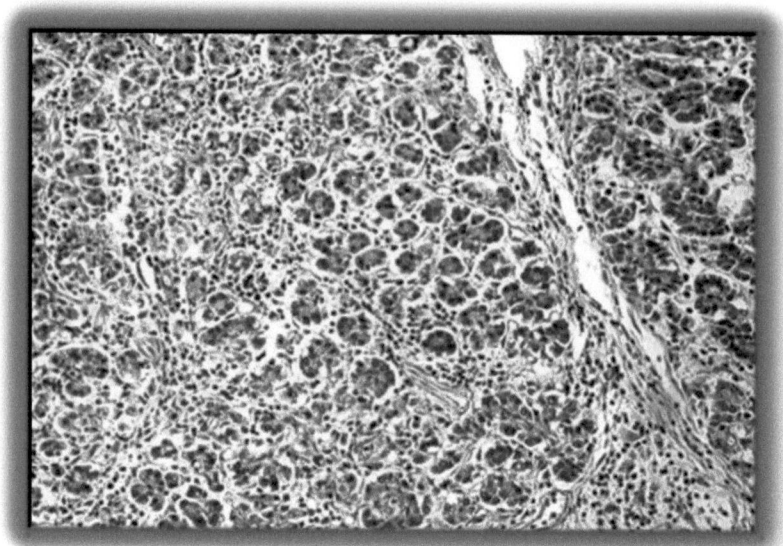

Figure 15 (HE 10x): Case 17. Presence of inflammatory infiltrate in interstitial site.

➢ Hemorrhage and edema (**Figure 16**). Fibrosis (**Figure 17**).

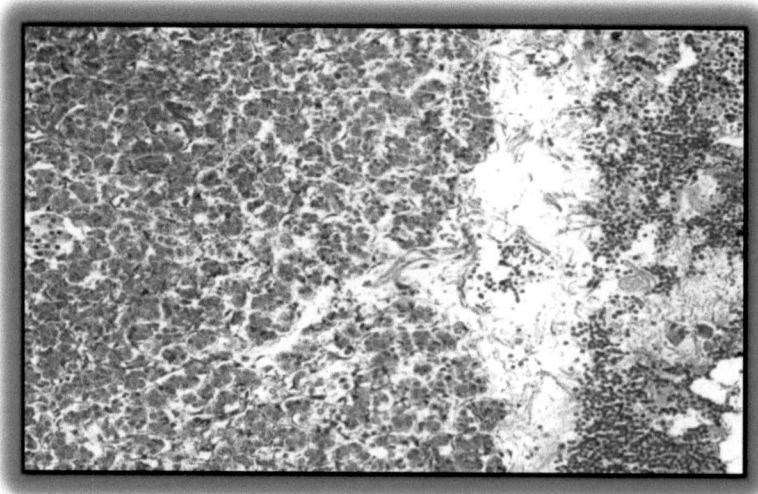

Figure 16 (HE 20x): Case 20. Recent hemorrhagic site and interstitial edema.

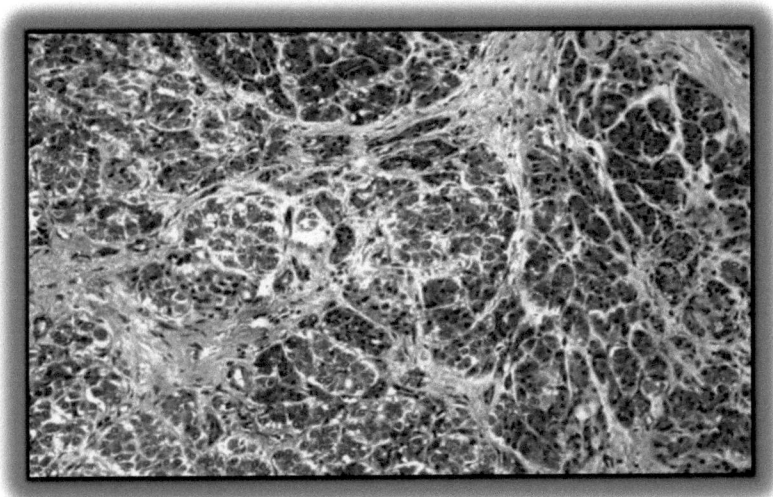

Figure 17 (Masson's trichrome 20x): Case 18. Presence of fibrous ridges characterized by the bluish coloration.

➤ Necrosis and abscesses (**Figure 18**). Granulomas (**Figure 19**).

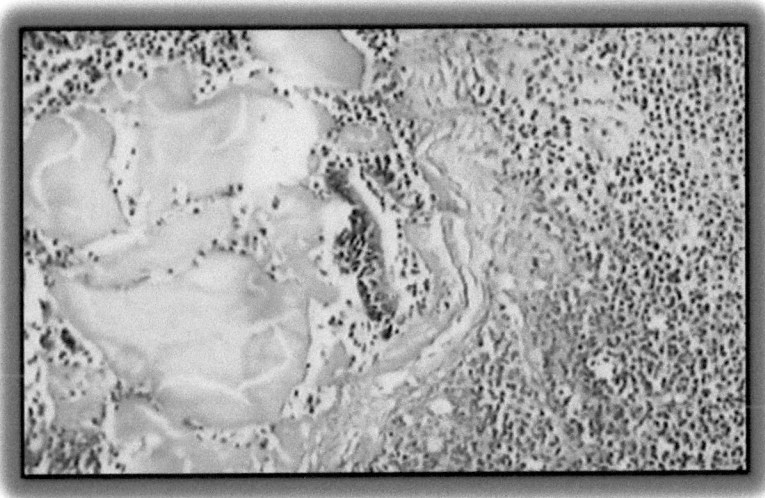

Figure 18 (HE 10x): Case 16. Presence of fat necrosis (steatonecrosis). Notice the presence of adjacent microabscess.

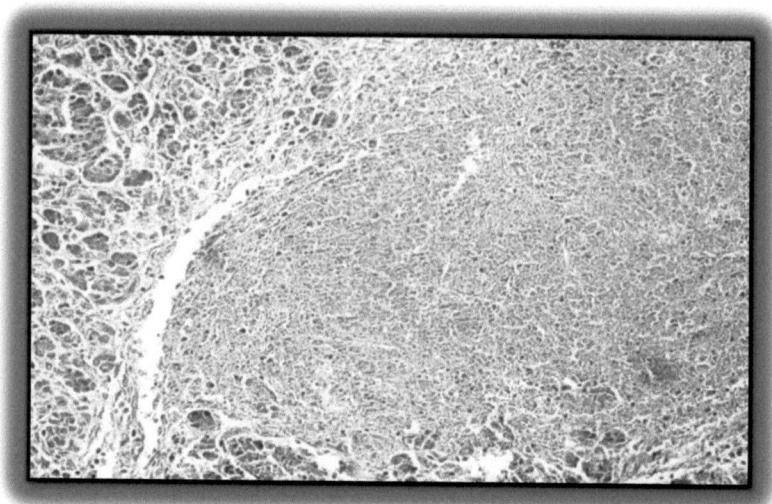

Figure 19 (HE 10x): Case 9. Caseous necrosis with granulomatous outline around it.

➢ Neoplasms (**Figures 20 and 21**)

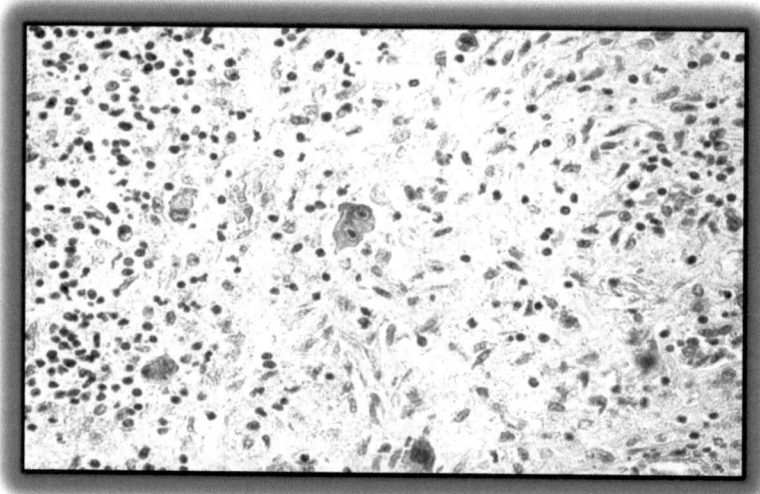

Figure 20 (HE 40X): Case 2. Hodgkin lymphoma characterized by the presence of Reed-Sternberg cell.

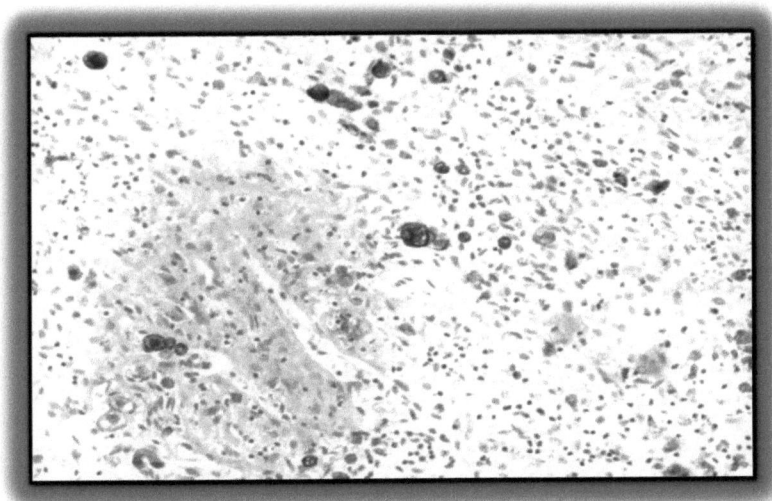

Figure 21 (Immunohistochemistry CD15 40x): Case 2. Hodgkin lymphoma. Positive CD15 in the Reed-Sternberg cell.

For fungal (**Figure 22**) and alcohol-acid resistant bacillus (AARB) (**Figure 23**) investigations, the histochemical techniques of SPA (Schiff's periodic acid) and Fite-Faraco were respectively used.

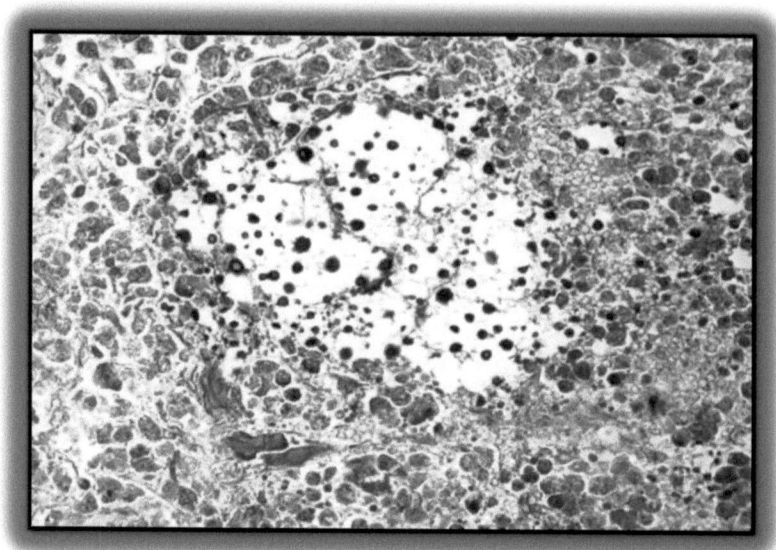

Figure 22 (SPA 40x): Case 16. Great amount of spores of *Cryptococcus sp.*

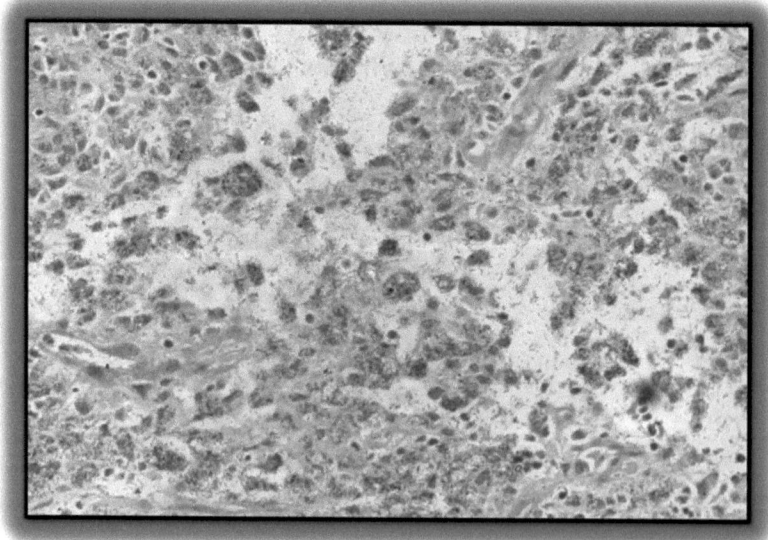

Figure 23 (Fite-Faraco 40x): Case 9. Numberless red-stained clustered AARB in the atypical mycobacteriosis.

13. DISCUSSION

The comparison of the data in relation to weight of the pancreas in Table 1 (anthropometric data and pancreatic parameters) showed that the groups are different. The HAART group presents pancreas weight values lower than the ones from the group without drugs, maybe a consequence of longer life expectancy and the possible effects of larger glandular depletion generated by the long use, malnutrition and the drug action that compromises the pancreas functioning.

In Table 2 (general clinical manifestations, alcoholism, smoking, pancreatic manifestations and drugs used in the treatment) it can be observed that fever occurred more frequently in the non-HAART group when compared to the HAART group, probably because the former did not make use of antiretroviral drugs and became more susceptible to opportunistic infections.

HIV-positive individuals develop two models of malnutrition: protein-caloric and wasting syndrome which cause fast and intense weight loss. Severe malnutrition reduces life expectancy and jeopardizes the quality of life in the HIV-positive patient.

Regarding the diarrhea described in Table 2, there were no significant differences between the two groups. The causes of diarrhea may be due to drug actions, changes in the intestinal luminal fluid tonicity, changes of the transport processes of electrolytes and water through the intestinal epithelium, undigested and unabsorbed nutrients because of the increase of the tonicity of the intestinal lumen in relation to the plasma, causing diarrhea of osmotic type and infectious processes by various pathogens [10,16,36,37].

In our sample, the side effects of antiretroviral drugs implied electrolyte imbalance and water absorptive process, a probable cause of diarrhea in the HAART group in relation to the non-HAART group.

The prevalence of increased abdominal pain in the HAART group may be associated with smoking and drinking, factors that were more frequent in the HAART group when compared with the non-HAART group. These are factors cause lesions such as chronic pancreatitis as well as pancreatic fibrosis.

Table 3A (semi-quantitative microscopic aspect of acinar components of the pancreatic stroma and histological aspects of acini) shows that the decrease of the zymogen granules, the decrease of nuclear dysplasia-like, the important increase of pancreatic atrophy, the increase of apoptosis and the maintenance of the parenchymal steatosis are more evident in the HAART group. These effects may be due to the longer life expectancy of HIV-positive individuals, and, as a result, the gland is in contact with the drugs, opportunistic agents and other damaging factors such as alcohol. With the reduction of the enzymes and atrophy of the parenchyma, we can assume that these patients may develop the malabsorption syndrome, represented by steatorrhea.

In the HAART group (Table 3B), another alteration was observed due to great abnormalities in the Langerhans islets represented by the increase in number, volume and dysplastic nuclei. These findings must be compatible to the longer use of antivirals.

Alterations in the Langerhans islets by a possible action of the antiretroviral therapy may decrease insulin secretion and glucose absorption by cells of the body as an energy source, increasing the concentration of glucose in the blood and thus causing diabetes. According to a study by Caseiro [38], it is reported that profound metabolic changes in HIV-positive patients are associated with the use of antiretroviral drugs like Stavudine, Indinavir and Lopinavir with Ritonavir. This mechanism can cause an alteration in insulin secretion in the HIV positive individual [38].

In Table 4 (acute pancreatitis, foci of lymphocytic inflammatory infiltrate and opportunistic infections detected at necropsy), foci of lymphocytic inflammatory infiltrate predominated in the HAART group owing to the irreversible irregular multifocal damage to the parenchymal gland. These infiltrates were caused by ductal alterations resulted from the pancreas necrotic inflammatory process. As a consequence, alterations in the exocrine and endocrine gland functions increase the number of diabetes cases, especially in the HAART group, probably due to the high rates of alcoholism.

Table 5 (immunohistochemical reactions for the characterization of infectious agents) shows that there were no significant differences concerning CMV (*Cytomegalovirus*) and PC (*Pneumocystis carinii*) infections in both groups.

When analyzing the last ten years of treatment for AIDS, it is remarkable how life expectancy has increased due to the introduction of the highly active antiretroviral therapy and its easy access to the general population. This is a fact that helped reduce death rates related to AIDS in 2010, justifying the sample of only 20 cases in the HAART group. The period to obtain 20 cases to accomplish this study was from June 2006 to December 2009. The samples obtained in 1995 encompassed 109 cases, probably due to a higher number of deaths (without potent antiviral therapy) and the unawareness of the disease and its consequences.

In this period of 15 years, the comparative casuistic analysis of the pancreas in 129 cases (109 cases in 1995 and 20 cases in 2010) was characterized by similarities of histological findings, ethnicity, and marital status, contrary to author's expectations. There was homogeneity among samples, despite the 15-year gap between groups.

The average age and a much higher incidence of the infection in males than in females in the HAART and non-HAART groups is in agreement with data supplied by the Ministry of Health and UNAIDS. This information came as a surprise, once AIDS epidemic has been turning to females. Nevertheless, the 2010 population is still predominantly composed of males and older individuals. This may be due to the fact the source of our patients was the Division of Postmortem Inspection of São Paulo, where autopsies are performed on patients who die suddenly, often without close monitoring in health centers and with poor adherence to antiretroviral treatment, or still, given the greater number of AIDS in males in Brazil. From 1980 to June 2010, there were 385,815 (65.1%) infection cases in males versus 207,080 (34.9%) in females according to the Bulletin of the Ministry of Health in 2010 [15]. The Bulletin actually bears records of the increasing rates of the disease among women, especially housewives. The Ministry of Health, however, now mentions the feminization of the epidemic in the country, since the difference between men and women has been shrinking. The number of cases in young people from 13 to 19 years of age increased, and this is the only age group in which the number of AIDS cases is higher among women [15].

The acquired immune deficiency syndrome and the pancreas in the HAART era were comparatively analyzed between HAART and non-HAART groups. It is important to highlight the fact that the HAART group shows a probable immunologic reconstitution with a significant decrease in the onset of opportunistic infections.

14. CONCLUSIONS

The analysis of the sample population of AIDS patients showed no differences between the two groups and the ones reported in other national and international centers regarding age, sex and race.

Concerning the macroscopic morphological aspects, there was a lower rate of pancreatic weight in the HAART group than in the non-HAART group. As to the findings in microscopic morphological aspects, highlighted in the histopathological pancreatic evaluation, the HAART group, when compared with the non-HAART group, showed a sharp decrease in zymogen granules, an increase in acinar atrophy, apoptosis, foci of lymphomononuclear inflammatory infiltrate and great alterations in the Langerhans islets.

The existence of a histopathologic pattern of pancreatic lesions, so common in AIDS after the use of antiretroviral therapy, could not be found.

15. REFERENCES

1. UNAIDS. Reporton the global AIDS epidemic 2010. [Internet]. [Updated 2011 Nov 06]. Available from: www.unaids.org/globalreport

2. Brazilian AIDS Bulletin 2010. Brazilian Health Ministry. [Internet]. [Updated 2011 Out 14]. Disponível a partir de www.aids.gov.br/sites/default/files/anexos/publicacao/2010/45974/boletim_dst_aids_2010_pdf_19557.pdf

3. Brivet F, Coffin B, Bedossa P, Naveau S, Petitpretz P, Delfraissy JF, et al. Pancreatic lesions in AIDS. *Lancet* 1987, **8558**:570-571.

4. Chehter EZ, Mott CB, Uip DE, Laudanna AA. AIDS and pancreas: a retrospective study. In: *10th World Congress of Gastroenterology*. Los Angeles: Abstract Book 1994. p. 587.

5. Chehter EZ. Acquired Immunodeficiency Syndrome (AIDS) and pancreas: a prospective study of clinical and pathological features. PhD tesis. Faculty of Medicine, USP. São Paulo, 1997.

6. Chehter EZ, Longo MA, Laudanna AA, Duarte MIS. Involvement of the pancreas in AIDS: a prospective study of 109 post-mortems. *AIDS* 2000, **14**: 1879-1886.

7. Balani AR, Grendell JH. Drug-Induced Pancreatitis. *Drug Safety* 2008, **3**(10): 823-837.

8. Riedel DJ, Gebo KA, Moore RD, Lucas GM. A Ten-Year Analysis of the Incidence and Risk Factors for Acute Pancreatitis Requiring Hospitalization in an Urban HIV Clinical Cohort. *AIDS Patient Care* STDS 2008, February **22**(2): 113-121.

9. Chehter EZ, Duarte MIS, Takakura CFH, Longo MA, Laudanna AA. Ultrastructural Study of the Pancreas in AIDS. *Pancreas* 2003, **26**(2):153-159.

10. Focaccia R, Veronesi R. Treaty of Infectious Diseases. In: *Gastrointestinal manifestations*. Part II. São Paulo: Atheneu; 2009. pp. 208-224.

11. Teixeira C, Gomes JRB, Gomes P, Maurel F. Viral surface glycoproteins gp120 and gp41, as potential targets against HIV-1: Brief overview one quarter of a century past the approval of zidovudine, the first ant-retroviral drug. In: *European Journal of Medicinal Chemistry* 2011, **46**:979-992.

12. Mincis M. Gastroenterology & Hepatology: diagnosis and treatment In: *Digestive Manifestations of Acquired Immunodeficiency Syndrome*. Mincis M (editor). São Paulo: Medical Reading; 2008. pp. 1172-1205.

13. Center for Disease Control and Prevention. Morbidity and Mortality Weekly Report. **MMWR**, 1994, **44**:64-68.

14. Klatt EC. **Pathology of AIDS**, version 21, Florida State University College of Medicine, mayor 27, 2011.

66**Nenhuma entrada de sumário foi encontrada.**15. Ministério da Saúde. **Boletim Epidemiológico – ADIS e DST**. [Internet]. [Updated 2010 Dezembro 8]. Disponível em: http://www.aids.gov.br/sites/default/files/anexos/publicacao/2010/45974/boletim_dst _aids_2010_pdf_19557.pdf

16. Robbins C. Pathological Basis of Disease. In: *The Gastrointestinal Tract*. Rio de Janeiro: Elsevier, 2005. p. 873-874.

17. Nadler, J. **Aids: etiopatogenia**. IN: *Focaccia R, Veronesi R*. Tratado de infectologia. 2 ed. São Paulo: Atheneu, 2004.

18. Riedel DJ, Gebo KA, Moore RD, Lucas GM. A ten-Year Analysis of the Incidence and Risk Factors for Acute Pancreatitis Requiring Hospitalization in an Urban HIV Clinical Cohort. In: *AIDS Patient care STDS*. 2008, **22(2)**:113-121.

19. Manfredi R, Calza L, Chiodo F. A Case-Control Study of HIV- Associated Pancreatic Abnormalities During HAART Era. Focus on Emerging Risk Factors and Specific Management. In: *Eur J Med Res*. 2004, **9**:537-544.

20. Junqueira, LC, Carneiro, J. Órgãos associados ao trato digestivo. In: *Histologia Básica*. 10ª ed. Rio de Janeiro, Brasil: Guanabara Koogan. 2004. pp. 317-338.

21. Brivet F, Coffin B, Bedossa P, Nauveau S, Petitpretz P, Delfraissy JF, Dormot, J. Pancreatic lesions. In: *AIDS*. Lancet 1987, **8558**:570-571.

22. Bricaine F, Marche C, Zoubi, Saimont AG, Renier B. HIV and the pancreas. In: *Lancet* 1988, **8575**:65-66.

23. Dowell, SF, Moore, GW, Hutchins GM. The spectrum of pancreatic pathology in patients with AIDS. Mod. *Pathol* 1990, **3**:49-53.

24. Bonacini M. Pancreatic involvement in human immunodeficiency virus infection. *J. Clin*. Gastroenterol 1991, **13**:58-64.

25. Chicarino JM, Cuzzi, T, Oliveira AV, Gutierrez GM, Cavalcanti RV, Grinsstejn, B, Tendrich M. Histopathologic findings in necropsy of endocrine glands in patients with AIDS. Int. Conf. *AIDS* 1992, **8**:112.

26. Klatt EC, Nichols L, Noguchi TT. Evolving trends revealed by autopsies of patients with acquired immunodeficiency syndrome. *Arch*. Pathol. Lab. Med 1994, **118**:884-90.

27. Cappell M. The pancreas in AIDS. *Gastroenterol Clin North Am*. 1997, **26**: 337-365.

28. Parentil DM, Steinberg W, Kang P. Infectious causes of acute pancreatitis. *Pancreas* 1996, **13**:356-71.

29. Carrocio A, Prima LDI, Grigoli CDI, Soresi C, Farinella E, Martino DDI, Guarino A, Notarbartolo A, Montalto. Exocrine Pancreatic Function and Fat Malabsorption in Human Immunodeficiency Virus-Infected Patients. *Scand J*. Gastroenterol 1999, **7**:729-734.

30. Carroccio A, Guarino A, Notarbartolo A, Montalto G, Fontana M, Zuin G, Montalto G, Canani RB, Verghi F, Bruzzese E. Efficacy of oral pancreatic enzyme theraphy for the treatment of fat Malabsorption in HIV-infected patients. *Aliment Pharmacol Ther* 2001, **15**:1619-1625.

31. Kerr JFR, Wyllie AH, Currie AR. APOPTOSIS: Abasic biological phenomenon with wide-ranging implications in tissue inetics. *BR J Cancer* 1972, **26**: 239-57.

32. Bradley EL. A clinically based classification system for acute pancreatitis: summary of the internacional symposium on acute pancreatitis. Atlanta 1992. *Arch Surg* 1993, **128**: 586-590.

33. Kloppell G, Maillet B. Pathology of acute and chronic pancreatitis. *Pancreas* 1993, **8**: 659-670

34. Michalany J. Technical histological pathology. Publisher Michalany; 1998; 3.

35. Stambulian M, Feliu S, Slobodianik NH. Nutritional status in patients with HIV infection and AIDS. *Br J Nutr*. 2007, **98 (Suppl 1)**:140-143.

36. Guyton AC. Treaty of Medical Physiology. In: *Physiology of the gastrointestinal disorders*. Rio de Janeiro: Elsevier; 2006.pp. 822-823.

37. Douglas CR. Treaty of Physiology applied to the medical sciences. In: *Physiology of the small intestine*. Rio de Janeiro: Guanabara Koogan; 2006.p. 934.

38. Caseiro MM. Alterações Metabólicas. [Internet]. [Updated 2012 May 15]. Disponível em: http://www.saberviver.org.br/index.php?g_edicao=alteracoes_metabolicas.

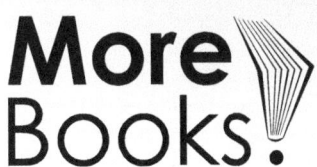
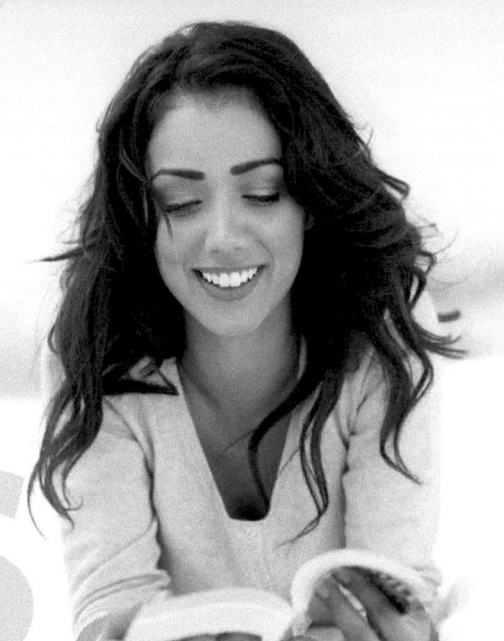

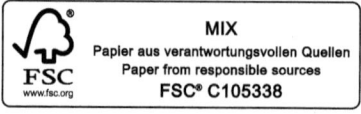

Printed by Books on Demand GmbH, Norderstedt / Germany